Department of Health and Social Security
Welsh Office
Scottish Home and Health Department

Immunisation against Infectious Disease

Joint Committee on Vaccination and Immunisation

London   Her Majesty's Stationery Office

© *Crown copyright 1988*
First published 1988

ISBN 0 11 321136 8

Preface

This edition of "Immunisation against Infectious Disease" represents a major revision of the previous handbook, and it is the wish of the Joint Committee that it will be updated annually. Its recommendations reflect the most recent advice available to the Joint Committee on Vaccination and Immunisation representing current expert medical opinion, although in some instances the recommendations may differ from those in the data sheets of the vaccine manufacturers.

The World Health Organisation has a stated aim in "Health for All" that by the year 2000, indigenous poliomyelitis, measles, neonatal tetanus, congenital rubella and diphtheria should have been eradicated from the European Region. This has the full support of my Committee.

No child should be denied immunisation without serious thought as to the consequences, both for the individual child and for the community.

We have been concerned that in the past children have been denied the benefits of vaccination because of the possibility of contraindications. We have attempted to deal with this, and have identified a number of false contraindications in the introduction and clarified the few which are genuine.

I would like to record my gratitude and that of my colleagues on the Joint Committee to Dr Christine Miller of the Public Health Laboratory Service and Dr David Salisbury of the Communicable Disease Division of the Department of Health and Social Security, for the great deal of time and effort they have put into this revision of the Memorandum.

SIR JOHN BADENOCH MA DM FRCP FRCP(Ed)
Chairman, Joint Committee on Vaccination and Immunisation
March 1988

The Joint Committee on Vaccination and Immunisation gratefully acknowledges the contributions to the Memorandum made by the BPA/JCVI Working Party, the Hepatitis Advisory Group, the BCG Subcommittee and the following individuals:–

Dr Joan Davies (Deputy Director, Public Health Laboratory Service)
Dr Sylvia Gardner (Virus Reference Laboratory, PHLS)
Dr David Magrath (Head of Biologics, WHO, and formerly National Institute for Biological Standards and Control)
Dr Elizabeth Miller (Communicable Disease Surveillance Centre, PHLS)
Dr Nigel Peel (Director, Leeds PHL)
Dr Frank Sheffield (David Bruce Laboratory, and formerly NIBSC)
Dr JWG Smith (Director, PHLS)
Professor Richard Smithells (Professor of Paediatrics and Child Health, University of Leeds)
Dr Bernard Rowe (Director, Division of Enteric Pathogens, PHLS)
Dr Susan Young (Deputy Director, CDSC).

Contents

			Page
Section	1	Introduction	1
	1.2	Preliminary Procedures	2
		Consent	2
		Contraindications	2
		HIV-positive persons	4
	2	Immunisation Procedures	7
		Nurses	8
		Anaphylaxis	9
		Schedule	11
	3	Whooping Cough	13
	4	Diphtheria	19
	5	Tetanus	25
	6	Poliomyelitis	30
	7	Measles	36
	8	Tuberculosis	42
	9	Rubella	52
	10	Measles/Mumps/Rubella	59
	11	Influenza	65
	12	Hepatitis B	70
		Hepatitis A	79
	13	Rabies	80
	14	Cholera	85
	15	Typhoid	89
	16	Anthrax	94
	17	Smallpox	97
	18	Yellow Fever	98
	19	Appendix: Immunoglobulin	111

1 Introduction

1.1.1 Immunity can be induced, either actively or passively, against a variety of bacterial and viral agents;

a. PASSIVE IMMUNITY results from injecting human immunoglobulin; the protection afforded is immediate but lasts only for a few weeks. Examples of its use are for protection of immuno suppressed children exposed to measles and for protection against hepatitis A and B (7.3.4, 12.8, 12.9 and Appendix).

b. ACTIVE IMMUNITY is induced by using inactivated or attenuated live organisms or their products. Examples of live attenuated vaccines include those for poliomyelitis (OPV), measles and rubella, and BCG vaccine. Other bacterial and viral vaccines such as whooping cough, typhoid and inactivated poliomyelitis (IPV) vaccines contain inactivated organisms. Others such as influenza and pneumococcal vaccine contain immunising components of the organisms; tetanus and diphtheria vaccines contain toxoid – that is, toxins inactivated by treatment with formaldehyde.

1.1.2 Most vaccines, apart from BCG, produce their protective effect by stimulating the production of antibodies which are detectable in the serum by laboratory tests. BCG vaccine promotes cell mediated immunity, identified by a positive tuberculin skin test. An important additional effect of poliomyelitis vaccine is the establishment of local immunity in the intestine.

1.1.3 A first injection of inactivated vaccine or toxoid in a subject without prior exposure to the antigen produces a slow antibody or antitoxin response of predominantly IgM antibody, the primary response. Two injections may be needed to produce such a response. Depending on the potency of the product and time interval, further injections will lead to an accelerated response in which the antibody or antitoxin titre (IgG) rises to a higher level – the secondary response. Following a full course, the antibody or antitoxin levels remain high for months or years, but even if the level of detectable antibody falls, the immune mechanism has been sensitised and a further dose of vaccine reinforces immunity.

1.1.4 Some inactivated vaccines contain adjuvants, substances which enhance the antibody response. Examples are aluminium phosphate and aluminium hydroxide which are contained in adsorbed diphtheria/tetanus/pertussis vaccine, and adsorbed diphtheria/tetanus vaccine.

1.1.5 Live attenuated virus vaccines such as measles, rubella and mumps promote a full, long-lasting antibody response after one dose. Live poliomyelitis vaccine (OPV) requires three doses.

1.2 Preliminary procedures

a. Consent must be obtained (1.2.1), and suitability for immunisation established.
b. Preparations must be made for the management of anaphylaxis and other immediate reactions.
c. Appropriate vaccination techniques must be known.

1.2.1 *Consent*
i) Consent must always be obtained before immunisation.
ii) Written consent provides a permanent record, but consent – either written or verbal – is required at the time of each immunisation after the child's fitness and suitability have been established (iv).
iii) Consent obtained before the occasion upon which a child is brought for immunisation is only an agreement for the child to be included in the immunisation programme.
iv) The bringing of a child to receive immunisation after an invitation to attend for this purpose may be viewed as acceptance that the child may be immunised. When a child is brought for this purpose and fitness and suitability have been established, consent to that immunisation may be implied in the absence of any expressed reservation to the immunisation proceeding at that stage.
v) If a child's fitness and suitability cannot be established, immunisation should be deferred.

1.2.2 *Contraindications*
a. Immunisation should be postponed if the subject is suffering from any acute illness. Minor infections without fever or systemic upset are not contra-indications.
b. Live vaccines should not be administered to pregnant women because of the theoretical possibility of harm to the fetus. However, where there is a significant risk of exposure, for example to poliomyeli-

tis or yellow fever, the need for vaccination outweighs any risk to the fetus.

c. Live vaccines should not be administered to the following: patients receiving high-dose corticosteroid (eg prednisolone 2mg/kg/day for more than a week), or immunosuppressive treatment including general irradiation; those suffering from malignant conditions such as lymphoma, leukaemia, Hodgkin's disease or other tumours of the reticuloendothelial system; patients with impaired immunological mechanism as for example in hypogammaglobulinaemia.

d. Children with immunosuppression from disease or therapy (eg in remission from acute leukaemia), should not receive live virus vaccines until at least six months after chemotherapy has finished. Such children and those in (c) above, should be given an injection of immunoglobulin as soon as possible after exposure to measles or chickenpox (see Appendix). NB. **Siblings and close contacts of such children must be immunised against measles.** Oral poliomyelitis vaccine (OPV) should not be given to these children, their siblings or other household contacts; inactivated poliomyelitis vaccine (IPV) should be used in its place. There is no risk of virus transmission following measles, mumps or rubella vaccines.

e. For children treated with systemic corticosteroids at high dose (eg prednisolone 2mg/kg/day for more than a week), live virus vaccines should be postponed until at least three months after treatment has stopped. Children on lower daily doses of systemic corticosteroids for less than two weeks, and those on lower doses on alternate day regimens for longer periods, may be given live virus vaccines.

f. Live virus vaccines, with the exception of yellow fever vaccine, should not be given within 3 months of an injection of immunoglobulin because the immune response may be inhibited. Normal human immunoglobulin obtained in the UK is unlikely to contain antibody to yellow fever virus which would inactivate the vaccine.

g. For HIV-positive individuals, see 1.3.

Contraindications to individual vaccines are listed in the relevant sections and must be observed.

1.2.3 The following conditions are NOT contraindications to vaccination:–

a. Asthma, eczema, hay fever or 'snuffles'.

b. Treatment with antibiotics or locally-acting (eg topical or inhaled) steroids.

Immunisation against Infectious Disease

c. Mother pregnant.
d. Child being breast fed.
e. History of jaundice after birth.
f. Under a certain weight.
g. Over the age given in immunisation schedule.
h. Previous history of pertussis, measles or rubella infection.
i. Prematurity: immunisation should not be postponed.
j. Stable neurological conditions such as cerebral palsy and Down's syndrome.

1.2.4 A history of allergy is NOT a contraindication. Hypersensitivity to egg contraindicates influenza vaccine; anaphylactic reaction to egg contraindicates measles and mumps vaccines.

1.2.5 *Special risk groups*
Some conditions increase the risk from infectious diseases and such children should be vaccinated as a matter of priority. These conditions include the following:– asthma, chronic lung and congenital heart disease, Down's syndrome, antibody- positive to the Human Immunodeficiency Virus (HIV, 1.3), small for dates and born prematurely. This last group should be immunised according to the recommended schedule from three months after birth, irrespective of the extent of prematurity.

1.2.6 If it is necessary to administer more than one live virus vaccine, they should either be given simultaneously in different sites (unless a combined preparation is used) or be separated by a period of at least three weeks. It is also recommended that a three week interval should be allowed between the administration of live virus vaccines and the giving of BCG.

1.3 *Immunisation of individuals with antibody to the Human Immunodeficiency Virus (HIV-positive)*
1.3.1 HIV-positive individuals WITH OR WITHOUT SYMPTOMS SHOULD receive the following as appropriate:–

Live vaccines: measles; mumps; rubella; polio.

Inactivated vaccines: whooping cough; diphtheria; tetanus; polio; typhoid; cholera; hepatitis B.

1.3.2 For HIV-positive symptomatic individuals, inactivated polio vaccine (IPV) may be used instead of OPV at the discretion of the clinician in charge.

1.3.3 HIV-positive individuals should NOT receive BCG vaccine; there have been reports of dissemination of BCG in HIV-positive individuals.

1.3.4 There is as yet insufficient evidence about the safety of use of yellow fever vaccine to allow recommendations to be made for HIV-positive asymptomatic individuals. It should not be given to symptomatic individuals.

1.3.5 No harmful effects have been reported following live attenuated vaccines for measles, mumps, rubella and polio in HIV-positive individuals who may be at increased risk from these diseases. It should be noted that in HIV-positive individuals, polio virus may be excreted for longer periods than in normal persons. Contacts of a recently vaccinated HIV-positive individual should be warned of this, and of the need for washing their hands after changing a vaccinated infant's nappies. For HIV-positive contacts of a vaccinated individual (whether that individual is HIV-positive or not) the potential risk of infection is greater than that in normal individuals.

1.3.6 Vaccine efficacy may be reduced compared with that in immuno-competent individuals. Consideration should be given to the use of normal immunoglobulin for HIV-positive individuals after exposure to measles.

1.3.7 For HIV-positive individuals exposed to chicken pox, see Immunoglobulin Section (Appendix).

NB. THE ABOVE ADVICE DIFFERS FROM THAT FOR OTHER IMMUNOCOMPROMISED PATIENTS (1.2.2)

1.3.5 For further information see: von Reyn CF, Clements CJ, Mann JM. Human Immunodeficiency Virus infection and routine childhood immunisation. Lancet 1987: ii: 669.

1.4 *Surveillance and reporting of suspected adverse reactions*
All vaccines are extensively tested for safety and efficacy but careful surveillance must be maintained. This depends on early, complete and

accurate reporting of suspected adverse reactions. It is essential that any abnormal clinical event following the administration of a vaccine should be reported on a yellow card without delay to the Committee on Safety of Medicines. Yellow cards are supplied to general practitioners and pharmacists, and are available from the Committee on Safety of Medicines, 1 Nine Elms Lane, London SW8 5NQ. They are also available as pages of the British National Formulary number 13 (1987) onwards.

1.5 Advice
No child should be denied immunisation without serious thought as to the consequences, both for the individual child and for the community. Where there is any doubt, advice should be sought from a Consultant Paediatrician, Specialist in Community Medicine or District Immunisation Coordinator.

2 Immunisation procedures

2.1 General

2.1.1 Before administering any immunological product, attention should be paid to the following points:
    a. The leaflets supplied with the product and prepared by the manufacturer in consultation with the Licensing Authority should be read (but see Preface).
    b. The identity of the vaccine must be checked to ensure the right product is used in the appropriate way on every occasion.
    c. The expiry date must be noted.
    d. The batch number must be recorded on the recipient's record.
    e. The recommended storage conditions must have been observed.

2.2 Reconstitution of vaccines

2.2.1 Freeze dried vaccines must be reconstituted with the diluent supplied and used within the recommended period after reconstitution. (See 2.7.2)

2.2.2 Before injection the colour of the product must be checked with that stated by the manufacturer in the package insert. The diluent should be added slowly to avoid frothing. A sterile 1 ml syringe with a 21G needle should be used for reconstituting the vaccine, and a small gauge needle for injection (see 2.8).

2.3 Cleaning of skin

2.3.1 The skin should be cleaned with a suitable preparation (eg mediswabs). Alcohol must be allowed to evaporate before injection of vaccine since it can inactivate live vaccine preparations.

2.4 Route of administration

    a. By mouth. Oral poliovaccine must NEVER be injected. Sugar lumps should be prepared with OPV immediately before administration; allowing them to stand at room temperature for any length of time may decrease the potency of the vaccine.

b. Subcutaneous and intramuscular injection.

With the exception of BCG, intramuscular or deep subcutaneous injection should be used for all vaccines. In infants, the antero-lateral aspect of the thigh or upper arm are recommended. If the buttock is used, injection into the upper outer quadrant avoids the risk of sciatic nerve damage, but injection into fatty tissue may reduce the efficacy of some vaccines.

c. Intradermal injection.

BCG vaccine is ALWAYS given intradermally; rabies vaccine may also be given this way. When giving an intradermal injection, the operator should stretch the skin between the thumb and forefinger of one hand, and with the other slowly insert the needle (size 25G), bevel upwards, for about 2mm into the superficial layers of the dermis, almost parallel with the surface. A raised, blanched bleb showing the tips of the hair follicles is a sign that the injection has been made correctly and its diameter gives a useful indication of the amount that has been injected. Considerable resistance is felt from a correctly given intradermal injection. If this is not felt, and it is suspected that the needle is too deep, it should be removed and reinserted before more vaccine is given. A bleb of 7mm diameter is approximately equivalent to 0.1ml.

d. Suitable sites for intradermal injections.

i) For BCG the site of injection is over the insertion of the left deltoid muscle; the tip of the shoulder must be avoided because of the increased risk of keloid formation at this site.

ii) For tuberculin sensitivity tests (Mantoux or Heaf), intradermal injections are given in the middle of the flexor surface of the forearm. This site should not be used for injecting vaccines.

iii) The use of jet injectors is NOT recommended.

iv) For intradermal rabies vaccine, the site of injection is behind the posterior border of the distal portion of the deltoid muscle.

2.5 Immunisation by nurses

A doctor may delegate responsibility for immunisation to a nurse provided the following conditions are fulfilled:

i) The nurse is willing to be professionally accountable for this work.

ii) The nurse has received training and is competent in all aspects of immunisation, including the contraindications to specific vaccines.
iii) Adequate training has been given in the recognition and treatment of anaphylaxis.

If these conditions are fulfilled and nurses carry out the immunisation in accordance with accepted District Health Authority policy, the Authority will accept responsibility for immunisation by nurses.

2.6 Anaphylaxis

Anaphylactic reactions are very rare, unexpected, and occasionally fatal. Any individual carrying out immunisation procedures must therefore be able to distinguish between anaphylaxis, convulsions, and fainting. The latter is relatively common after immunisation of adults and adolescents; very young children rarely faint and sudden loss of consciousness at this age should be presumed to be an anaphylactic reaction in the absence of a strong central pulse (ie carotid) which persists during a faint or convulsion.

The following signs and symptoms may develop:
i) Pallor, limpness and apnoea are the commonest signs in children.
ii) Upper airway obstruction; hoarseness and stridor as a result of angio-oedema involving hypopharynx, epiglottis and larynx.
iii) Lower airway obstruction; subjective feelings of retrosternal tightness and dyspnoea with audible expiratory wheeze from bronchospasm.
iv) Cardiovascular; sinus tachycardia, profound hypotension in association with tachycardia; severe bradycardia.
v) Skin; characteristic rapid development of urticarial lesions – circumscribed, intensely itchy weals with erythematous raised edges and pale blanched centres.

Management
Such events happen without warning. Appropriate emergency equipment must therefore be immediately at hand whenever immunisation is given. All doctors and nurses responsible for immunisation must be familiar with the practical steps necessary to save life following an anaphylactic reaction.
i) Lie patient in left lateral position. If unconscious, insert airway.

ii) Give 1/1000 adrenaline by deep intramuscular injection unless there is a strong central pulse and the patient's condition is good. See Table below for dosage.
iii) If oxygen is available, give it by face mask.
iv) Send for professional assistance. NEVER LEAVE PATIENT ALONE.
v) If appropriate, begin cardio-pulmonary resuscitation.
vi) At the doctor's discretion, hydrocortisone 100mg and/or chlorpheniramine maleate (piriton) 2.5–5mg may be given intravenously.
vii) If there is no improvement in the patient's condition in 10 minutes, repeat the dose of adrenaline up to a maximum of 3 doses.
viii) All cases should be admitted to hospital for observation.
ix) The reaction should be reported to the Committee on Safety of Medicines using the yellow card system.

Adrenaline dosage Adrenalin 1/1000 (1mg/ml)
Adults: 0.5 to 1.0 ml repeated as necessary up to a maximum of 3 doses. The lower dose should be used for the elderly or those of slight build.

Infants and children:

Age	Dose of adrenaline
Less than 1 year	0.05ml
1 year	0.1ml
2 years	0.2ml
3–4 years	0.3ml
5 years	0.4ml
6–10 years	0.5ml

2.7 Storage of vaccine

2.7.1 Manufacturers' recommendations on storage must be observed. No vaccines must be kept at temperatures below 0°C as freezing can cause deterioration of the vaccine and breakage of the container.

2.7.2 Reconstituted vaccine must be used within the recommended period, varying from one to four hours, according to the manufacturer's instructions. Single dose containers are preferable; once opened, multi-dose vials must not be kept after the end of the session and any vaccine left unused must be discarded.

2.8 Administration

Vaccine	Route of administration	Dose	Needle size
OPV	Oral	3 drops	Nil
IPV	Deep subcutaneous or intramuscular	0.5ml	23 G
DPT) DT)	Deep subcutaneous or intramuscular	0.5ml	23 G
Measles) Mumps) Rubella)	Deep subcutaneous or intramuscular	0.5ml	23 G
Typhoid	Deep subcutaneous or intramuscular	0.5ml	23 G
BCG	Intradermal Infants	0.1ml 0.05ml	25 G
Rabies	Deep subcutaneous or intramuscular Intradermal	1.0ml 0.1ml	23 G 25G
Anthrax	Deep subcutaneous or intramuscular	0.5ml	23 G
Hepatitis B	Deep subcutaneous or intramuscular	1.0ml	23 G

2.8.1 *Immunoglobulin*. See Appendix

2.9 Schedule

The schedule for routine immunisation, with the recommended ages and intervals between doses, is given below. Details of procedure for each vaccine are given in the relevant sections and should be consulted.

While the ages recommended are those considered to be the most effective for each vaccine, every effort should be made to ensure that all children are vaccinated even if they present outside the recommended age-range. No opportunity to vaccinate should be missed.

Immunisation Procedures

Vaccine	Age		Notes
	Primary course		
D/T/P and polio	1st dose	3 months	For accelerated schedule see 3.3.2
	2nd dose	4½–5 months	
	3rd dose	8½–11 months	
Measles	12–18 months		Can be given at any age over 12 months
Measles/mumps/ rubella from 1.10.88	12–18 months		As for measles
D/T and polio	4–5 years		
Rubella	10–14 years		
BCG	10–14 years		Interval of 3 weeks between BCG and rubella
Tetanus and polio	15–18 years		

CHILDREN should therefore have received the following vaccines:

By end of first year: 3 doses of DTP and polio, or DT and polio.
By end of second year: measles. (MMR from 1.10.88).
By school entry: 4th DT and polio; measles or MMR if missed earlier.
Between 10 and 14 years: BCG and rubella.
Before leaving school: 5th polio and tetanus.

ADULTS should receive the following:

Women sero-negative for rubella: rubella vaccine.
Previous unimmunised individuals: polio vaccine; tetanus vaccine.
Individuals in high risk groups: hepatitis B vaccine; influenza vaccine.

3 Whooping Cough

3.1 Introduction

3.1.1 Whooping cough is a highly infectious bacterial disease caused by *Bordetella pertussis* and spread by droplet infection; the incubation period is 7 to 10 days. It is infectious from 7 days after exposure to three weeks after the onset of typical paroxysms. The initial catarrhal stage has an insidious onset and is the most infectious period. An irritating cough gradually becomes paroxysmal, usually within 1–2 weeks, and often lasts for 2–3 months. In young infants, the typical "whoop" may never develop and coughing spasms may be followed by periods of apnoea. Whooping cough may be complicated by bronchopneumonia, repeated post-tussive vomiting leading to weight loss, and by cerebral hypoxia with an attendent risk of brain damage. Severe complications and deaths occur most commonly in infants under 6 months of age who can be protected only by immunisation of their older siblings.

3.1.2 Before the introduction of whooping cough vaccination in 1957 the average annual number of notifications exceeded 100,000. By 1973, when vaccine acceptance was over 80%, annual notifications of whooping cough had fallen to around 2,400.

3.1.3 Because of public anxiety about the safety and efficacy of the vaccine, acceptance fell to about 30% in 1975 and major epidemics followed in 1977/79 and 1981/83. However the return of public confidence which led to increased vaccine acceptance (67% in 1986) stopped the next epidemic which died away in 1986 well below the levels of the previous two. Notifications remained low throughout 1987.

3.1.4 Until the mid 1970s, mortality from whooping cough was about 1 per 1000 notified cases with a higher rate for infants under 1 year. In 1978 however when there were over 65,000 notifications, only 12 deaths were notified. The actual number of deaths due to whooping cough is undoubtedly higher since not all cases in infants are recognised.

3.1.5 Since the anxieties in the mid 1970s concerning whooping cough vaccine, studies have confirmed that a full course of vaccine confers protection in over 80% of recipients; in those not fully protected the disease is usually less severe. The two large epidemics which followed the reduction in vaccine acceptance are additional evidence of the effectiveness of whooping cough vaccine in the prevention of disease. In Regions with particularly low vaccine acceptance rates, whooping cough notifications in 1977–79 were significantly higher than those in Regions where acceptance was higher than the national average.

3.2 Vaccine

3.2.1 Whooping cough vaccine is a suspension of killed *Bordetella pertussis* organisms with an estimated potency of not less than 4 International Units in each 0.5ml of vaccine. The vaccine is usually given as a triple vaccine combined with diphtheria and tetanus vaccines, with an adjuvant such as aluminium hydroxide (DTPer/Vac/Ads, Trivax Ads). It is also available without the adjuvant as plain DTPer/Vac, and as a monovalent pertussis vaccine. The adsorbed vaccine should be used as it is more immunogenic and causes fewer systemic reactions, especially fever.

3.2.2 Adsorbed diphtheria/tetanus/pertussis vaccine (DTPer/Vac/Ads): one 0.5ml dose consists of a mixture in isotonic saline of diphtheria toxoid and tetanus toxoid adsorbed on to aluminium hydroxide gel, together with not more than 20,000 million *Bordetella pertussis* organisms. The potency of the diphtheria component is not less than 30 IU; that of the tetanus component not less than 40 IU and that of the whooping cough component not less than an estimated 4 IU. Thiomersal is added as a preservative to a final concentration of 0.01 per cent.

3.2.3 Monovalent pertussis vaccine: one 0.5ml dose contains not more than 20,000 million *Bordetella pertussis* organisms. Thiomersal is added as a preservative to a final concentration of 0.01 per cent.

The vaccines should be stored between 2–8°C, but not frozen. 0.5ml should be given by deep subcutaneous or intramuscular injection.

3.3 Recommendations

3.3.1 Adsorbed whooping cough vaccine as a component of the primary course of immunisation against diphtheria, tetanus and whooping cough (DTPer/Vac/Ads) is recommended for all infants from 3 months of age, unless there is a genuine contra indication (see 3.5).

3.3.2 The primary course consists of three doses with an interval of 6–8 weeks between the first and second, and 4–6 months between the second and third. If whooping cough is prevalent, the interval between doses can be reduced to four weeks. If the primary course is interrupted it should be resumed but not repeated, allowing appropriate intervals between the remaining doses.

3.3.3 Monovalent whooping cough vaccine can be used when the whooping cough component has been omitted from earlier vaccinations. Children who have received a full course of vaccination against diphtheria and tetanus should be given 3 doses of monovalent whooping cough vaccine at monthly intervals.

3.3.4 Where the primary course of diphtheria/tetanus immunisation has been started and the parent agrees, triple vaccine may be used to complete it, followed by monovalent whooping cough vaccine at monthly intervals. Similarly, children presenting for their pre-school diphtheria/tetanus booster who have not previously been immunised against whooping cough should be given triple vaccine as the first dose, and the course completed with monovalent whooping cough vaccine at monthly intervals. There is no contraindication to the vaccination of unimmunised older children against whooping cough in order to protect infants and siblings. There is no upper age limit. No reinforcing dose of whooping cough vaccine is necessary after a course of three injections.

3.3.5 If whooping cough vaccine is contraindicated or refused by parents, then DT/Vac/Ads should be offered.

3.3.6 HIV-positive individuals may receive whooping cough vaccine in the absence of contraindications given in 3.5.

3.4 Adverse Reactions

3.4.1 a. A small painless nodule may form at the injection site which usually disappears and is of no consequence.
 b. Crying, screaming and fever may occur after whooping cough

vaccine in triple vaccine; they may also occur after vaccine which does not contain the whooping cough component. Attacks of high pitched screaming, episodes of pallor, cyanosis, limpness, convulsions, as well as local reactions have been reported with similar frequency after both adsorbed vaccines; both local and systemic reactions are more common after the plain preparation which does not contain adjuvant.

c. Neurological events including convulsions and encephalopathy may very rarely occur after whooping cough vaccine. The best estimate of risk to an apparently normal infant of suffering neurological reaction such as a prolonged febrile convulsion after whooping cough vaccine is about one in 100,000 injections, almost all of these occurring without permanent consequence. Neurological complications after whooping cough disease are considerably more common than after immunisation. However in both immunised and unimmunised children, encephalopathy resulting in permanent brain damage or death may occur in the first year of life; no wholly reliable estimate of the risk of such complications after whooping cough vaccine can therefore be made. There is no specific test to identify those cases of encephalopathy which may be due to whooping cough vaccine.

3.4.2 When pertussis vaccine is contraindicated, an infant should still be considered for immunisation against diphtheria and tetanus.

3.4.3 If a febrile convulsion occurs after a dose of triple vaccine, specialist advice should be sought before continuing with any immunisation.

3.4.4 Severe reactions to whooping cough vaccine must be reported to the Committee on Safety of Medicines, using the yellow card system.

3.5 Contraindications to Whooping Cough immunisation

3.5.1 a. If the child is suffering from any acute illness immunisation should be postponed until it has fully recovered. Minor infections without fever or systemic upset should be ignored.

b. Immunisation should not be carried out in children who have a history of severe local or general reaction to a preceding dose. The following reactions should be regarded as severe:–
Local: an extensive area of redness and swelling which becomes indurated and involves most of the antero-lateral surface of the thigh

or a major part of the circumference of the upper arm. This reaction may increase in severity with each subsequent injection.

General: fever equal to or more than 39.5°C within 48 hours of vaccine; anaphylaxis; bronchospasm; laryngeal oedema; generalised collapse; prolonged unresponsiveness; prolonged inconsolable screaming; convulsions occurring within 72 hours.

3.6 A personal or family history of allergy is NOT a contraindication to immunisation against whooping cough, nor are stable neurological conditions such as cerebral palsy or spina bifida. For other false "contraindications" see 1.2.3.

3.7 Children with problem histories

There are certain groups of children in whom the advisability of whooping cough immunisation requires special consideration because of their own or their family histories. For these, the risk from vaccine may be higher, but the effects of whooping cough disease could be more severe. The balance of risk and benefit should be assessed in each case. Where there is doubt, appropriate advice should be sought from a consultant paediatrician or specialist in community medicine before a decision is made to withhold vaccine.

These groups are:
  i)   Children with a documented history of cerebral damage in the neonatal period;
  ii) Children with a personal history of convulsions;
  iii) Children whose parents or siblings have a history of idiopathic epilepsy. In such children there may be a risk of developing a similar condition irrespective of vaccine.

3.8 Management of Outbreaks

Since a course of 3 injections is required to protect against whooping cough, vaccine cannot be used to control an outbreak. However, intervals between injections may be reduced to one month (see 3.3.2).

Immunisation against Infectious Disease

3.9 Supplies

All whooping cough vaccines are manufactured and supplied by the Wellcome Foundation Ltd. Tel. Crewe (0270) 583151.

3.10 Bibliography

DHSS Whooping Cough: Reports from the Committee on Safety of Medicines and the Joint Committee on Vaccination and Immunisation. HMSO 1981.

Miller CL and Fletcher WB
Severity of notified whooping cough
BMJ 1976, (1), 117–119.

Miller DL, Ross EM, Alderslade R, Bellman MH, Rawson NSB
Pertussis immunisation and serious acute neurological illness in children
BMJ 1981, 282, 1595–1599.

Nelson KB and Ellenberg JH
Prognosis in children with febrile seizures
Paediatrics 1978, 61, 720–727.

Pollock TM, Miller E, Mortimer JY, Smith G
Symptoms after primary immunisation with DTP and with DT vaccine
Lancet 1984, 146–149.

PHLS Epidemiological Research Laboratory and 21 Area Health Authorities
Efficacy of pertussis vaccination in England
BMJ 1982, 285, 357–359.

Pollard R
Relation between vaccination and notification rates for whooping cough in England and Wales
Lancet 1980, i, 1180–82.

4 Diphtheria

4.1 Introduction

4.1.1 Diphtheria is now a rare acute infectious disease affecting the upper respiratory tract and occasionally the skin. It is characterised by an inflammatory exudate which forms a greyish membrane in the respiratory tract which may cause obstruction. The incubation period is from 2 to 5 days. The disease is communicable for up to 4 weeks, but carriers may shed organisms for longer. A toxin is produced by diphtheria bacilli which affects particularly myocardium and nervous and adrenal tissues. Spread is by droplet infection and through contact with articles soiled by infected persons (fomites).

4.1.2 Effective protection against the disease is provided by active immunisation. The introduction of immunisation against diphtheria on a national scale in 1940 resulted in a dramatic fall in the number of notified cases and deaths from the disease. In 1940, 46,281 cases with 2,480 deaths were notified, compared with 37 cases and 6 deaths in 1957. From 1979 to 1986, 26 cases were notified with only 1 death. The disease and the organism have been virtually eliminated from the United Kingdom and there is now no possibility of natural immunisation from sub-clinical infection. Thus a high vaccine acceptance rate must be maintained in order to protect the population against the possibility of a resurgence of the disease which could follow the introduction of cases from overseas.

4.2 Diphtheria vaccine

4.2.1 Diphtheria immunisation protects by stimulating the production of antitoxin which provides immunity to the effects of the toxin. The immunogen is prepared by treating a cell-free purified preparation of toxin with formaldehyde, thereby converting it into the innocuous diphtheria toxoid. This however is a relatively poor immunogen, and for use as a vaccine it is usually adsorbed on to an adjuvant, either aluminium phosphate or aluminium hydroxide. *Bordetella pertussis* also acts as an effective adjuvant.

4.2.2 The vaccines available are:

Adsorbed vaccines:

Diphtheria/tetanus/pertussis
Diphtheria/tetanus
Diphtheria
Diphtheria vaccine for adults (low dose)

Plain vaccines:

Diphtheria/tetanus/pertussis
Diphtheria/tetanus

Vaccines should be stored at 2–8°C. The dose is 0.5ml given by intramuscular or deep subcutaneous injection.

4.3 Recommendations

4.3.1 For immunisation of infants and children under 10 years.
 a. Primary immunisation.
Diphtheria vaccine as a component of triple vaccine (diphtheria toxoid, tetanus toxoid and *Bordetella pertus: is*) is recommended for infants from 3 months old. Adsorbed vaccine should be used as it has been shown to cause fewer reactions than plain vaccine. If the pertussis component is contraindicated, adsorbed diphtheria/tetanus vaccine should be used. A course of primary immunisation consists of 3 doses with an interval of 6–8 weeks between first and second doses, and 4–6 months between the second and third doses. If a course is interrupted it may be resumed; there is no need to start again.
 b. Reinforcing immunisation
A dose of vaccine containing diphtheria and tetanus toxoids is recommended for children immediately before school entry, preferably after at least 3 years from the last dose of the primary course.

4.3.2 Immunisation of persons aged 10 years or over.
 a. Primary immunisation.
Diphtheria vaccine for adults (low dose) MUST be used. Three doses of 0.5ml should be given by deep subcutaneous or intramuscular injection at intervals of 1 month.
 b. Reinforcing immunisation.
A single dose of 0.5ml is required. This low-dose diphtheria vaccine MUST be used for all persons aged 10 years and over; prior Schick testing is not necessary.

4.3.3 Contacts of a diphtheria case, or carriers.

Individuals exposed to such a risk should be given a complete course or a reinforcing dose according to their age and immunisation history as follows:
  a. Immunised children under 10 years.
One injection of diphtheria vaccine.
  b. Immunised children over 10 years, and adults.
One injection of diphtheria vaccine for adults (low dose).
  c. Unimmunised children under 10 years.
Three injections of diphtheria vaccine as described in 4.3.1.
  d. Unimmunised children over 10 years, and adults.
Three injections of diphtheria vaccine for adults (low dose), as described in 4.3.2.

Unimmunised contacts of a case of diphtheria should in addition be given a prophylactic course of erythromycin.

4.3.4 HIV-positive individuals may be immunised against diphtheria in the absence of any contra indications (4.7).

4.4 Use of the Schick test

4.4.1 The Schick test is recommended for individuals who may be exposed to diphtheria in the course of their work. In such cases immunity to diphtheria should be ensured by means of a Schick test carried out at least three months after immunisation is completed.

4.5 Schick test

4.5.1 An intradermal injection of 0.2ml of Schick test toxin is given into the flexor surface of the left forearm and 0.2ml of Schick test control (inactivated toxin) material into the corresponding position of the right forearm, using separate syringes and needles. Readings should be made at 24–48 hours and 5–7 days. Comparison of the appearance of the two injection sites will reveal responses attributable to immunity and to allergy. Four types of response may occur:
  a. Schick negative.
No visible reaction on either arm. The subject is IMMUNE and need

not be immunised or reinforced.

    b. Schick positive.

An erythematous reaction develops at the site of the toxin injection, becoming evident in 24–48 hours and persisting for 7 days or more before gradually fading. The control shows no reaction. The subject is NOT IMMUNE and requires to be immunised or reinforced.

    c. Negative-and-pseudo-reaction.

Both injection sites show similar reactions after 48–72 hours, which fade within 5–6 days. The reactions are due to hypersensitivity to the components of the test materials. The subject is IMMUNE and need NOT be immunised or reinforced.

    d. Positive-and-pseudo-reaction (also called combined reaction).

Both injection sites show reactions after 48–72 hours but the reaction in the LEFT arm (toxin) is usually larger and more intense than that on the RIGHT arm. The control response fades considerably by the 5th–7th day leaving the positive effect clearly evident. Such combined reactors usually have a basal immunity to diphtheria and should NOT be immunised with a further full course of vaccine. Their immunity can successfully be reinforced by a single injection of diphtheria vaccine for adults (low-dose).

4.6 Adverse reactions

4.6.1 Transient fever, headache, malaise and local reactions may occur. A small painless nodule may form at the injection site but usually disappears without sequelae. Severe anaphylactic reactions are rare. Neurological reactions have been reported occasionally.

4.6.2 Severe reactions should be reported to the Committee on Safety of Medicines using the yellow card system.

4.7 Contraindications

See Sections 1.2.2 and 1.2.3 of Introduction.

4.7.1 Diphtheria vaccination is elective except when there is a need to control an outbreak. It should not be given to anyone suffering from an acute febrile illness unless diphtheria is suspected. Low-dose diphtheria vaccine for adults MUST be used for persons aged 10 years and over.

4.8 Diphtheria antitoxin

4.8.1 Diphtheria antitoxin is now only used in suspected cases of diphtheria. Tests with a trial dose to exclude hypersensitivity should precede its use. It should be given without waiting for bacteriological confirmation since its action is specific for diphtheria. It may be given intramuscularly or intravenously, the dosage depending on the clinical condition of the patient. It is no longer used for diphtheria prophylaxis because of the risk of provoking a hypersensitivity reaction to the horse serum from which it is derived. Unimmunised contacts of a case of diphtheria should be promptly investigated, kept under surveillance and given antibiotic prophylaxis and vaccine as in 4.3.3.

4.9 Supplies

4.9.1 Diphtheria vaccines (4.2.2) EXCEPT low-dose diphtheria vaccine for adults are manufactured and supplied by Wellcome Foundation Ltd. Tel. 0270 583151. ADSORBED VACCINE MUST BE SPECIFIED OR PLAIN VACCINE WILL BE SUPPLIED.

4.9.2. Low-dose diphtheria vaccine for adults is manufactured by Swiss Serum and Vaccine Institute, Berne, and distributed in the UK by Regent Laboratories Ltd, Cunard Road, London NW10 6PN. Tel. 01-965 3637.

4.9.3 Schick Test Toxin and Schick Test Control BP. Manufactured and supplied by Wellcome Foundation Ltd. Tel. 0270 583151.

4.9.4 Diphtheria antitoxin is supplied in vials containing 2000 IU per ml. Manufactured by the Swiss Serum and Vaccine Institute, Berne, and distributed in the UK by Regent Laboratories Ltd, Cunard Road, London NW10 6PN. Tel. 01-965 3637.

4.10 Bibliography

Anderson A
Some observations on diphtheria immunisation
The Medical Officer 1957, 97, 161–163.

Diphtheria

Bainton D, Freeman M, Magrath D, Sheffield FW, Smith JGW
Immunity of children to diphtheria, tetanus and poliomyelitis
BMJ 1979, (1), 854–857.

Butler NR, Voyce MA, Burland WL, Hilton ML
Advantages of aluminium hydroxide adsorbed combined diphtheria, tetanus and pertussis vaccines for the immunisation of infants
BMJ 1959, (1), 663–666.

Report of Ad Hoc Working Group
Susceptibility to diphtheria
Lancet 1978, (i), 428–430.

Sheffield FW, Ironside AG, Abbot JD
Immunisation of adults against diphtheria
BMJ 1978, (2), 249–250.

5 Tetanus

5.1 Introduction

5.1.1 Tetanus is an acute disease characterised by muscular rigidity with superimposed agonising contractions. It is induced by the toxin of tetanus bacilli which grow anaerobically at the site of an injury. The incubation period is between 4 and 21 days, commonly about 10. Tetanus spores are present in soil and may be introduced into the body during injury, often a puncture wound, but also through burns or trivial, unnoticed wounds. Tetanus neonatorum due to infection of the baby's umbilical stump is an important cause of death in many countries of Asia, Africa and South America. World-wide elimination of neonatal tetanus by the year 2000 is one of the WHO targets. Tetanus is not spread from person to person.

5.1.2 Effective protection against tetanus is provided by active immunisation. This was introduced routinely as part of the primary immunisation of infants in 1961. From 1960–1969 there were approximately 27 annual deaths in England and Wales in which tetanus was implicated. In 1970 it was recommended in the UK that active immunisation should be universal and that in the treatment of wounds, active immunity to tetanus should be initiated and subsequently completed.

5.1.3 In the 1970s around 20 cases of tetanus were notified annually, probably about a third of the actual number. From 1974–8 there were 22 deaths assigned to tetanus with a further 21 in which tetanus was present. From 1981–86 there were 62 notifications, with only 3 cases in children under 15 years of age, and 25 in persons aged 65 years and over. Tetanus is thus increasingly a disease of the older age groups who did not receive routine primary immunisation in childhood or during service in the armed forces.

5.2 Tetanus vaccine and adsorbed Tetanus vaccine

5.2.1. Immunisation protects by stimulating the production of antitoxin which provides immunity against the effects of the toxin. The immunogen is prepared by treating a cell-free preparation of toxin with formaldehyde and thereby converting it into the innocuous tetanus toxoid.

The vaccines available for immunisation are:

Adsorbed vaccines:

Tetanus
Diphtheria/tetanus
Diphtheria/tetanus/pertussis

Plain vaccines:

Tetanus
Diphtheria/tetanus
Diphtheria/tetanus/pertussis

Vaccines should be stored at 2–8°C. The dose is 0.5ml given by intramuscular or deep subcutaneous injection.

5.3 Recommendations

5.3.1 For immunisation of infants and children under 10 years.
  a. Primary immunisation.
Triple vaccine, that is, vaccine containing diphtheria toxoid, tetanus toxoid, and *Bordetella pertussis*, is recommended for infants from 3 months of age. Either adsorbed or plain vaccine may be used but adsorbed is preferable as it has been shown to cause fewer reactions. If the pertussis component is contraindicated adsorbed diphtheria/tetanus vaccine should be used. A course of primary immunisation consists of 3 doses with an interval of 6–8 weeks between the first and second doses and 4–6 months between the second and third doses. If a course is interrupted it may be resumed; there is no need to start again. The dose is 0.5ml given by intramuscular or deep subcutaneous injection.
  b. Reinforcing doses in children
Diphtheria/tetanus vaccine is recommended immediately prior to school entry, preferably with an interval of at least 3 years from the last dose of the primary course. A further reinforcing dose of tetanus vaccine alone is recommended for those aged 15–19 years or before leaving school.

5.3.2 For immunisation of adults and children over 10 years.
  a. For primary immunisation the course consists of 3 doses of 0.5ml by intramuscular or deep subcutaneous injection, with intervals of 6–8

weeks between the first and second and 4–6 months between the second and third.

  b. A reinforcing dose 5 years after the primary course and again 10 years later maintains a satisfactory level of protection.

5.3.3 *For treatment of patients with tetanus prone wounds*
Emergency treatment is required for patients with wounds in the following categories:

  a. Any wound or burn sustained more than six hours before surgical treatment.

  b. Any wound or burn at any interval after injury that shows one or more of the following characteristics:
    i) a significant degree of devitalised tissue
    ii) puncture-type wound
    iii) direct contact with soil or material likely to harbour tetanus organisms
    iv) clinical evidence of sepsis

Whatever the tetanus immunisation history of the patient, a thorough surgical toilet of the wound is essential. Specific anti-tetanus treatment must be given as follows:

Patients who are NOT KNOWN to have been fully immunised against tetanus.
Antitetanus immunoglobulin by intramuscular injection in one limb (see Appendix 19.3.1), and the first of a course of 3 injections of adsorbed tetanus vaccine in another. The remaining 2 injections must be given at monthly intervals.

Patients who completed a primary course or received a reinforcing dose MORE THAN 10 YEARS PREVIOUSLY.
One injection each of antitetanus immunoglobulin and adsorbed tetanus vaccine.

Patients who completed a primary course or received a reinforcing dose WITHIN 5–10 YEARS.
One dose of adsorbed tetanus vaccine.

Patients who completed a primary course or received a reinforcing dose WITHIN 5 YEARS.
These may be considered immune and not in need of treatment. However if it is considered that there is a high risk of tetanus, a single dose of vaccine may be given.

NB. Routine tetanus immunisation began in 1961, and thus individuals born before that year will not have been immunised in infancy. A full course of immunisation may be required unless it has previously been given, as for instance in the armed services. Antitetanus immunoglobulin is rarely required for patients already immunised against tetanus, bcause in such individuals adequate protection can be achieved by giving a single injection of adsorbed tetanus vaccine.

5.3.4 For wounds not in the above categories, such as clean cuts, immunoglobulin should NOT be given.

5.3.5 Patients with impaired immunity may not respond to vaccine and may therefore require additional tetanus immunoglobulin (see Appendix 19.3.1) for wounds listed in 5.3.3.

5.3.6 HIV-positive individuals should be immunised against tetanus in the absence of contraindications (5.5).

5.4 Adverse reactions

5.4.1 Local reactions, such as pain, redness and swelling round the injection site may occur and persist for several days. General reactions, which are uncommon, include headache, lethargy, malaise, myalgia and pyrexia. Acute anaphylactic reactions and urticaria may occasionally occur and, rarely, peripheral neuropathy. Persistent nodules at the injection site may arise if the injection is not given deeply enough.

5.4.2 Severe reactions should be reported to the Committee on Safety of Medicines using the yellow card system.

5.5 Contraindications

See Sections 1.2.2 and 1.2.3 of Introduction.

5.5.1 Reinforcing doses of tetanus vaccine at less than 5 year intervals may provoke hypersensitivity reactions and should be avoided. Tetanus vaccine should not be given if the patient is suffering from acute febrile illness except in the presence of a tetanus-prone wound.

5.6 Supplies

5.6.1 All DTP and DT vaccines manufactured by and available from Wellcome Foundation Ltd, Crewe. Tel. 0270 583151. Adsorbed tetanus vaccine also available from: Evans Medical. Tel. 0582 608308; Merieux UK Ltd. Tel. 0628 785291.

5.6.2 Antitetanus immunoglobulin: Blood Product Laboratory. Tel. 01-953 6191; Wellcome (Humotet) see above.

5.7 Bibliography

Bainton D, Freeman M, Magrath DI, Sheffield F, Smith JWG
Immunity of children to diphtheria, tetanus and poliomyelitis
BMJ 1979, (i), 854–857.

Edsall G, Elliott MW, Peebles TC, Levine L, Eldred MC
Excessive use of tetanus toxoid boosters
JAMA 1967, 202 (i), 17–19.

White WG et al
Duration of immunity after active immunisation against tetanus
Lancet 1969, (ii) 95–96

White WG
Reactions after plain and adsorbed tetanus vaccines
Lancet 1980, (i), 42

Sheffield FW
To give or not to give; guidelines for tetanus vaccine
Community View 1985, 33, 8–9

Smith JWG, Lawrence DR, Evans DG
Prevention of tetanus in the wounded
BMJ 1975, (iii), 453–455.

6 Poliomyelitis

6.1 Introduction

6.1.1 Poliomyelitis is an acute illness following invasion of the gastro-intestinal tract by one of the three types of poliovirus (I, II and III). The virus has a high affinity for nervous tissue and the primary changes are in neurones. The infection may be clinically inapparent, or range in severity from a non-paralytic fever to aseptic meningitis or paralysis. Symptoms include headache, gastro-intestinal disturbance, malaise and stiffness of the neck and back, with or without paralysis. The infection rate in households with young children can reach 100%. The proportion of inapparent to paralytic infections may be as high as 1000 to 1 in children and 75 to 1 in adults, depending on the poliovirus type and the social conditions. Poliomyelitis remains endemic in some developing countries where it occurs in epidemics. In countries with an effective immunisation programme the disease occurs as sporadic cases, or in outbreaks amongst unvaccinated individuals. Transmission is through contact with the faeces or pharyngeal secretions of an infected person.

6.1.2 The incubation period ranges from 3 to 21 days. Cases are most infectious from 7 to 10 days before and after the onset of symptoms; virus may be shed in the faeces for up to 6 weeks or longer.

6.1.3 Inactivated poliomyelitis vaccine (Salk) was introduced in 1956 for routine vaccination, and was replaced by attenuated live oral vaccine (Sabin) in 1962. Individuals born before 1956 may not have been immunised and no opportunity should be missed to immunise them in adult life. Since the introduction of vaccine, notifications of paralytic poliomyelitis have dropped from nearly 4,000 in 1955 to a total of 35 cases between 1974–1978. This included 25 cases during 1976 and 1977, in which infection with wild virus occurred in unvaccinated persons, demonstrating the continuing need to maintain high levels of vaccination uptake. Since 1979 notifications have averaged 3 per year, nearly every case being either imported or vaccine associated.

6.2 Poliomyelitis vaccine (live and inactivated)

a. Live oral poliovaccine (OPV) is routinely used for immunisation in the UK, always given by mouth. It contains live attenuated strains of poliomyelitis virus types I, II and III grown in cultures of monkey kidney cells or on human diploid cells. The attenuated viruses become established in the intestine and promote antibody formation both in the blood and the gut epithelium, providing local resistance to subsequent infection with wild poliomyelitis viruses. This reduces the frequency of symptomless excretion of wild poliomyelitis virus in the community. OPV inhibits simultaneous infection by wild polioviruses and is thus of value in the control of epidemics. Vaccine strain poliomyelitis virus may persist in the faeces for up to 6 weeks after OPV. Whilst a single dose may give protection, a course of three doses produces a long-lasting immunity to all 3 poliovirus types.

OPV should be stored at 0–4°C, and the expiry date should be checked before use. Vaccine stored unopened at 0–4°C is stable, but once the containers are open it may lose its potency. Any vaccine remaining in opened containers at the end of an immunisation session must therefore be discarded.

b. Inactivated poliovaccine (IPV) contains polioviruses of all three types inactivated by formaldehyde. It should be stored at 0–4°C. 0.5ml is given by deep subcutaneous or intramuscular injection (6.3.5). A course of 3 injections produces long-lasting immunity to all 3 poliovirus types.

6.3 Recommendations

6.3.1 *Primary immunisation of infants and children*
Oral poliovaccine is recommended for infants from 3 months of age. The primary course consists of 3 separate doses with intervals of 6–8 weeks between the first and second dose, and 4–6 months between the second and third doses, given at the same time as diphtheria/tetanus/pertussis vaccine. In infants the dose of 3 drops of vaccine is dropped from a spoon directly into the mouth, whilst in children it is given on a sugar lump. The dose should be repeated if the vaccine is regurgitated.

Breast-feeding does not interfere with the antibody response to OPV and immunisation should not be delayed on this account. Faecal excretion of vaccine virus may lead to infection of unimmunised contacts; usually such infection is of no consequence, but see 6.4. The contacts of a recently vaccinated baby should be advised of the need for strict personal hygiene, particularly for washing their hands after changing the baby's napkins.

6.3.2 *Reinforcing immunisation in children*
A reinforcing dose of oral poliomyelitis vaccine (OPV) should be given before school entry at the same time as the reinforcing dose of diphtheria and tetanus vaccine; a further dose of OPV should be given at 15–19 years of age before leaving school.

6.3.3 *Immunisation of adults*
A course of three doses of OPV at intervals of 4 weeks is recommended for the primary immunisation of adults. No adult should remain unimmunised against poliomyelitis (see 6.1.3).

Reinforcing doses for adults are not necessary unless they are at special risk, such as:
    a. travellers to countries where poliomyelitis is epidemic or endemic. (See "The Traveller's Guide to Health – Before You Go" SA 40, 1988.)
    b. health care workers in possible contact with poliomyelitis cases.

6.3.4 For those exposed to a continuing risk of infection a single reinforcing dose is desirable every 10 years.

6.3.5 Inactivated poliovaccine (IPV) is available for the immunisation of individuals for whom a live vaccine is contraindicated (see 1.2.2d). It should also be used for siblings and other household contacts of immuno suppressed individuals. A primary course of three doses of 0.5ml should be given by deep subcutaneous or intramuscular injection with the same time intervals as for OPV. Reinforcing doses should be given as for OPV.

6.3.6 HIV-positive individuals may receive live polio vaccine but excretion of the vaccine virus in the faeces may continue for longer than in normal individuals. Household contacts should be warned of this and for the need for hand-washing after nappy changes.

6.3.7 For HIV-positive symptomatic individuals, IPV may be used instead of OPV at the discretion of the clinician in charge.

6.4 Adverse reactions

6.4.1 Cases of vaccine-associated poliomyelitis have been reported in recipients of OPV and in contacts of recipients. In England and Wales there is an annual average of one recipient and one contact case in relation to over 2 million doses of oral vaccine. Contact cases would be eliminated if all children and adults were vaccinated. The possibility of a very small risk of poliomyelitis induced by OPV cannot be ignored but is insufficient to warrant a change in vaccination policy.

6.4.2 Severe reactions following immunisation with poliomyelitis vaccine (6.4.1) should be reported to the Committee on Safety of Medicines using the yellow card system.

6.5 Contraindications

See Sections 1.2.2 and 1.2.3 of Introduction.
   a. Febrile illness; immunisation should be postponed.
   b. Vomiting or diarrhoea.
   c. Treatment involving high-dose corticosteroids or immuno-suppression including general radiation (see 1.2.2d).
   d. Malignant conditions such as lymphoma, leukaemia, Hodgkin's disease and other tumours of the reticuloendothelial system and where the normal immunological mechanism may be impaired as for example, in hypogammaglobulinaemia. See also 1.2.2d.
   e. Although adverse effects on the fetus have not been reported, oral poliovaccine should not be given to women during the first 4 months of pregnancy unless there are compelling reasons.

6.5.2. OPV may be given at the same time as inactivated vaccines and with other live virus vaccines. If not given simultaneously with other live virus vaccines, an interval of three weeks should be observed; this also applies to BCG vaccine.

6.5.3 Both OPV and IPV may contain trace amounts of penicillin and streptomycin but these do not contraindicate their use except in extreme cases of hypersensitivity. Both vaccines contain neomycin in small amounts and OPV may also contain polymyxin.

6.5.4 OPV should NOT be used for the siblings and other household contacts of immunosuppressed children; such contacts should be given IPV.

6.5.5 OPV should be given either 3 weeks before or 3 months after an injection of normal immunoglobulin (12.9.3). This may not always be possible in the case of travellers abroad, but as in such cases the OPV is likely to be a booster dose the possible inhibiting effect of immunoglobulin is less important.

6.6 Management of outbreaks

6.6.1 After a single case of paralytic poliomyelitis, a dose of OPV should be given to all persons in the immediate neighbourhood of the case (with the exception of people suffering from immunodeficiency), regardless of a previous history of immunisation against poliomyelitis. In previously unimmunised individuals the course must be completed. If there is laboratory confirmation that a vaccine-derived poliovirus is responsible for the case, vaccination of further possible contacts is unnecessary since no outbreaks associated with vaccine virus have been documented to date. If the source of the outbreak is uncertain, it should be assumed to be a "wild" virus and appropriate control measures instituted.

6.7 Supplies

6.7.1 a. Oral poliomyelitis vaccine is available in 10 × 1 dose packs and in dropper tubes of 10 doses from Wellcome Foundation (Tel. 0270 583151) and Smith Kline and French Ltd (Tel. 0707 325111).
 b. Inactivated poliovaccine (IPV) is supplied in single dose 1ml ampoules. Manufactured by Smith, Kline and French Limited. Obtained from DHSS, 14 Russell Square, London WC18 5EP (Tel. 01-636 6811) or from Welsh Office, Greyfriars Road, Cardiff.

6.8 Bibliography

Collingham KE, Pollock TM, Roebuck MO

Paralytic poliomyelitis in England and Wales 1976–77
Lancet 1978, (i), 976–977.

John TJ et al
Effect of breast feeding on sero-response of infants to oral poliovaccine
Pediatrics 1976, 57, 47–53.

Begg NT, Chamberlain R, Roebuck M
Paralytic poliomyelitis in England and Wales 1970–84
Epidem Inf 1987, 99, 97–106.

Bainton D, Freeman M, Magrath DI, et al
Immunity of children to diphtheria, tetanus and poliomyelitis
BMJ 1979, (i), 854–857.

Roebuck M, Chamberlain R
Prevalence of antibodies to poliovirus in 1978 among subjects aged 0–88 years
BMJ 1982, 284, 697–700

White P, Green J
Prevalence of antibody to poliovirus in England and Wales 1984–6
BMJ 1986, 293, 1153–1155.

7 Measles

7.1 Introduction

7.1.1 Measles is an acute viral illness transmitted via droplet infection. Clinical features include Koplik spots, coryza, conjunctivitis, bronchitis, skin rash and fever. The incubation period is about 10 days, with a further 4 days before the rash appears. It is highly infectious from the beginning of the prodromal period to 4 days after the appearance of the rash. Complications have been reported in 1 in 15 notified cases, and include otitis media, bronchitis, pneumonia, convulsions, and encephalitis, which has an incidence of 1 in 5000 cases. Electroencephalographic changes have been reported after apparently uncomplicated measles as well as in cases with frank encephalitis. Complications are more common and severe in poorly nourished and chronically ill children and it is therefore particularly important that such children should be immunised against measles.

7.1.2 Notification of measles began in England and Wales in 1940, and until the introduction of vaccine in 1968 annual notifications varied between 160,000 and 800,000, the peaks occurring in two year cycles. By the mid-seventies notifications had fallen to between 50,000 and 180,000 and the biennial pattern had disappeared. Deaths from measles declined from 1000 in 1940 to 90 in 1968 and the decline has continued since the introduction of vaccination, to an annual average of 13 deaths in the period 1970–1986. More than half the deaths were in previously healthy unvaccinated children, the majority of whom were over the age at which vaccine is given. Between 1970 and 1983, 19 children aged between 2 and 8 years who were in remission from acute lymphatic leukaemia died from measles. An additional average of 10 deaths a year result from subacute sclerosing panencephalitis, a rare but inevitably fatal complication of measles infection.

7.1.3 From 1968 to 1980 measles vaccine acceptance for children aged 1–2 years remained between 50% and 60%. By 1986 the overall figure had increased to 71%, but acceptance in individual Districts varied between 29% and 89%.

7.2 Measles vaccine

7.2.1 Measles vaccine is a freeze-dried preparation containing live attenuated measles virus. (Attenuvax, Mevilin-L, Rimevax). It must be stored in the dried state at 2–8°C (NOT frozen) and reconstituted immediately before use with the diluent fluid supplied by the manufacturer. A single dose of 0.5ml is given by deep subcutaneous or intramuscular injection. Vaccination results in sero-conversion in 95% of recipients. Vaccine-induced antibody titres tend to be lower than those following natural infection, but have nevertheless been shown to persist for at least 15 years. The attenuated vaccine virus is not transmitted and there is thus no risk of infectivity.

7.3 Recommendations

7.3.1 Measles vaccine should be given to ALL children aged 1 to 2 years for whom there is no valid contraindication (7.5). Since measles is still most common between 1 and 4 years, vaccination is most effective shortly after the first birthday. It should not be given below the age of 12 months because it is ineffective in the presence of maternal antibody which may persist to that age. It has been shown that a history of "measles" under 2 years is not confirmed by the presence of antibody; such a history should thus be ignored and the child vaccinated.

7.3.2 If immunisation has been missed at 1–2 years it can be given at any age, and no opportunity should be missed to ensure that this is done. If the primary course of DTP and polio immunisation has not been completed at the time that measles vaccine is due, both can be given at the same time using a separate syringe and different sites. Similarly, if children who attend for pre-school immunisation (D/T/polio) have not received measles vaccine, it should be given then.

7.3.3 Unimmunised children in the following groups are at particular risk from measles infection and SHOULD be vaccinated:
   a. children with chronic conditions such as cystic fibrosis, congenital heart or kidney disease, failure to thrive, Down's syndrome.
   b. children from the age of one year upwards in residential or day care, including playgroups and nursery schools.

Measles

7.3.4 Children with compromised immunity (7.5a and b) who come into contact with measles should be given normal immunoglobulin as soon as possible after exposure (see Appendix 19.2.1). Children under 12 months in whom there is a particular reason to avoid measles (such as recent severe illness), can also be given immunoglobulin; the latter should then be given measles vaccine after an interval of at least 3 months, at around the usual age.

7.3.5 As vaccine-induced antibody develops more rapidly than that following natural infection, vaccination can be used to protect susceptible contacts. To be effective the vaccine must be administered within three days of exposure.

7.3.6 Revaccination is only necessary when vaccine has been given before 12 months of age.

7.3.7 Children with a personal history of convulsions, or whose parents or siblings have a history of idiopathic epilepsy, SHOULD receive measles vaccine. It should be given to such children after their parents have been given advice for prophylactic treatment against febrile convulsions.

7.3.8 Measles immunisation of adults is unnecessary since very few are still susceptible to measles, but there is no upper age limit. Vaccine should be considered for young adults in long-term institutional care who may not have acquired immunity.

7.3.9 HIV-positive individuals may be given measles vaccine in the absence of contraindications (7.5).

7.4 Adverse reactions

7.4.1 Adverse reactions to measles vaccine are few when compared with the incidence of complications of natural measles. The most common reactions are malaise and fever, with or without rash, occurring 5–10 days after vaccination. These seldom last more than 48 hours and the vaccine virus is not transmitted. Febrile convulsions may occur in a very small proportion of children, particularly if there is a coincidental infection. The incidence of convulsions following measles infection in children aged 1–2 is 8 to 10 times higher than that following vaccine.

7.4.2 Encephalitis is a rare complication of measles vaccination and, as with febrile convulsions, has a much higher incidence following measles infection.

7.4.3 Allergic reactions to measles vaccine may occur very occasionally. (See Anaphylaxis, 2.6.)

7.4.4 Severe reactions following measles vaccine should be reported to the Committee on Safety of Medicines using the Yellow Card system.

7.5 Contraindications

See Sections 1.2.2 and 1.2.3 of Introduction.

7.5.1 Vaccination should be postponed in individuals suffering from a febrile illness. It must not be given to the following:
   a. patients receiving corticosteroid or immunosuppressive treatment, including general irradiation;
   b. patients suffering from malignant diseases such as lymphoma, leukaemia, Hodgkin's disease or other tumours of the reticuloendothelial system, or where the normal immunological mechanism may be impaired as in hypogammaglobulinaemia;
   c. pregnant women, because of the theoretical risk of fetal infection.
   d. measles vaccine should not be given within 3 months of an injection of immunoglobulin.

7.5.2 If it is necessary to give more than one live virus vaccine, the vaccines should be given simultaneously at different sites (unless a combined preparation is used), or be separated by an interval of at least 3 weeks. A 3-week interval should also be allowed between live virus vaccines and BCG.

7.5.3 Measles vaccine should not be given to persons known to be hypersensitive to neomycin or polymyxin. The vaccine does not contain penicillin. Allergy to hens' eggs is no longer considered to be a contraindication to the vaccine, except in individuals with a history of anaphylactoid reactions to egg ingestion (generalised urticaria, swelling of the mouth and throat, difficulty in breathing, hypotension and shock) who should not be given measles vaccine. Dislike of egg and allergy to chicken feathers are not contraindications. For other false contraindications to vaccination, see Introduction, 1.2.3.

7.5.4 Measles virus inhibits the response to tuberculin, so tuberculin-positive individuals may become tuberculin-negative for up to a month after measles infection or immunisation. Because the measles virus may cause exacerbation of tuberculosis, such patients should be under treatment when immunised.

7.6 Management of outbreaks

7.6.1 The spread of measles can be contained by giving vaccine to susceptible children within 72 hours of their being in contact with a case. If there is doubt about a child's measles immunity, vaccine should be given, since there are no ill-effects from giving vaccine to those already immune. Human normal immunoglobulin is available for individuals for whom vaccine is contraindicated (Appendix 19.2.1).

7.7 Supplies

7.7.1 The following live attenuated measles vaccines (Meas/Vac(Live)) are available:

Mevilin L (Schwarz strain) Evans Medical (Tel. 0582 608308); Rimevax (Schwarz strain) Smith Kline and French (Tel. 0707 325111); Attenuvax (Enders Edmonston strain) Morson (Tel. 0992 467272).

7.7.2 For supplies of immunoglobulin, see 7.3.7 and Appendix.

7.8 Bibliography

Miller DL
Frequency of complications of measles 1963
BMJ 1964, (II). 75–78.

Miller CL
Severity of notified measles
BMJ 1978, (i), 1253.

Miller CL
Deaths from measles
BMJ 1985, 290, 443–444.

Adjaye N, Azad A, Foster M, Marshall WC, Dunn H
Measles serology in children with a history of measles in early life.
BMJ 1983, 286, 1478.

Buynak E, Weibal RE, et al
Long-term persistence of antibody following Enders' original and more attenuated live measles virus vaccine
Proc Soc Exp Biol Med 1976, 153, 441–443.

Miller CL
Live measles vaccine: a 21 year follow up
BMJ 1987, 295, 22–24.

Herman JJ, Radin R, Schneiderman BS
Allergic reactions to measles (rubeola) vaccine in patients hypersensitive to egg protein
J Pediatrics, 1983, 102, 2, 196–9.

Lingam S, Miller CL, et al
Antibody response and clinical reactions in children given measles vaccine with immunoglobulin
BMJ 1986, 292, 1044–5.

8 Tuberculosis: BCG Vaccination

8.1 Introduction

8.1.1 Tuberculosis is caused by *Mycobacterium tuberculosis* or *Mycobacterium bovis* and may affect any part of the body, but infection is usually acquired via the respiratory route. The incidence of the disease has declined over the years (although it is higher in Scotland than in England and Wales) but the case-fatality rate remains above 10%. When considering BCG vaccination, particular attention should be given to immigrants from developing countries and to those travelling to high-risk areas.

8.2 Bacillus Calmette-Guerin (BCG) vaccine (intradermal)

8.2.1 BCG vaccine (intradermal) contains a live attenuated strain derived from *Mycobacterium bovis*. It is supplied freeze-dried, with diluent in a separate ampoule, and is available free of charge from the Supply Division of the appropriate Health Department. Surveys in British school children have shown that the vaccine is over 70% effective with protection lasting at least 15 years.

8.2.2 BCG vaccine should be stored at 2–8°C and protected from light. It should not be used after the expiry date stated on the label. The ampoule should be opened using suitable aseptic precautions and the contents should be used within one hour of reconstitution and in any case should not be kept longer than the one session.

8.3 Vaccination

8.3.1 The dose of BCG vaccine is 0.1ml injected intradermally (reduced to 0.05ml for infants under 3 months of age). The use of a separate needle and syringe for each patient is essential to avoid the risk of transmission of hepatitis etc. The injection must be given strictly intradermally and not subcutaneously. The site of inoculation should be at the insertion of the deltoid muscle as sites higher on the arm are more likely to lead to keloid formation. The tip of the shoulder should be avoided. In girls, for cosmetic reasons, the upper and lateral surface of the thigh may be preferred. Apart from newly-born babies, any person who is being considered for BCG vaccination should first have a skin test for hypersensitivity to tuberculoprotein.

8.3.2 Before giving an intradermal injection, the skin should be swabbed with spirit and allowed to dry. When giving an intradermal injection the operator should stretch the skin between thumb and forefinger of one hand and with the other slowly insert the needle, with the bevel upwards, for about 2mm into the superficial layers of the dermis almost parallel with the surface. The needle should be short, with a short bevel which can usually be seen through the epidermis during insertion. A raised blanched bleb showing the tips of the hair follicles is a sign that the injection has been made correctly and its diameter gives a useful indication of the amount that has been injected. A bleb of 7mm diameter is approximately equivalent to 0.1ml injection.

8.3.3 Considerable resistance is felt from a correctly given intradermal injection; if this is not felt and it is suspected that the needle is too deep, it should be removed and reinserted before more vaccine is given.

8.4 Groups for which BCG vaccination is recommended

8.4.1 It is recommended that these groups be vaccinated if found negative for tuberculoprotein hypersensitivity:
   a. Contacts of cases known to be suffering from active respiratory tuberculosis. The children of immigrants in whose communities there is a high incidence of tuberculosis may for this purpose be regarded as contacts. Newly-born babies who are contacts need not be tested for sensitivity but should be vaccinated without delay.
   b. Health service staff: this category should include medical students, hospital medical staff, nurses, and anybody who comes into contact with patients, including physiotherapists and radiographers, technical staff in pathology departments and any others considered to be at special risk because of the likelihood of contact with infective patients or their sputum. It is particularly important to test staff working in maternity and paediatric departments.
   c. School children between the ages of 10 and 13 years.
   d. Students including those in teacher training colleges.

8.4.2 After inoculation with BCG vaccine there is a high conversion rate and only staff who have a high risk of contact with tuberculous patients and tuberculous pathological material need further observation. Staff in this high risk group should have the site of vaccination inspected six weeks after inoculation to confirm that a satisfactory reaction has occurred. Only those who show no evidence of a reaction require a post-BCG skin test, after which those who are tuberculin negative should be re-vaccinated. If there is still no evidence of a satisfactory reaction or conversion to a positive tuberculin test, they should be employed elsewhere in the Health Service where they are unlikely to be exposed to tuberculosis. They must not handle tuberculous material until found to be tuberculin positive or have demonstrated a satisfactory reaction to vaccination. The normal time to carry out a post-vaccination test is 6–12 weeks after vaccination.

8.4.3 BCG vaccination of infants is normally recommended where:
  i) the infant is known to be a contact of a case of active respiratory tuberculosis;
  ii) the infant belongs to an immigrant community characterised by a high incidence of tuberculosis;
  iii) the infant will reside in or travel to any area where the risk of tuberculosis is judged to be high or where crowded living conditions exist.

Vaccination may be carried out soon after birth and newly-born babies, even if contacts, need not be tested for sensitivity beforehand. Otherwise infants may be vaccinated at any age following skin-testing although BCG must not be administered within three weeks of any live virus vaccine. The dose of BCG is reduced to 0.05ml for infants under 3 months. Special care must be taken to ensure that the injection is made intradermally. As for adults, a separate syringe and needle must be used for each infant. *Jet injectors should not be used.*

8.5 Testing for hypersensitivity to tuberculoprotein (tuberculin skin testing)

8.5.1 Hypersensitivity testing techniques
Except for newly-born babies, this test should always be undertaken when BCG vaccination is contemplated, to assess the individual's sensitivity to tuberculoprotein. To ensure uniformity of results it is

desirable to use the official supply of purified protein derivative (PPD) which is available, free of charge, from the appropriate Health Department. Care must be taken that the correct preparation of PPD is used for skin-testing (see footnote). It is recommended that one of the two well-established methods described below should be used.

8.5.2 All tuberculin PPD must be stored between 2–8°C (never frozen) and protected from light. Once an ampoule is opened, its contents should be used within an hour and not retained beyond the one session.

8.5.3 Nurses or health visitors specially trained in the techniques involved and working under the supervision of an experienced doctor may be employed to perform the sensitivity skin tests and to read and record the results.

8.5.4 *The intradermal test (Mantoux test)*
An area of skin, over the upper third of the flexor surface of the forearm, is cleaned with spirit and 0.1ml of tuberculin PPD dilution 100 units/ml is injected intradermally so that a wheal is produced of about 7 mm in diameter. A separate needle and syringe must be used for each patient. The results should be read after 72 hours but usually a valid reading can be obtained up to 96 hours. A positive result consists of induration at least 6mm diameter.

FOOTNOTE: Tuberculin Purified Protein Derivative (PPD) BP is a sterile preparation made from the heat-treated products of growth and lysis of the appropriate mycobacterium at a strength of 100,000 units/ml. This strength is however only used for the Heaf test and three dilutions of PPD are available for other skin tests. It is very important that the correct strength is used:

Strength units/ml	Dilution PPD	Units in dose of 0.1ml	Main use
1,000	1 in 100	100	* see below
100	1 in 1,000	10	Mantoux test (routine)
10	1 in 10,000	1	Mantoux test (special)

* this dilution is only used for special diagnostic purposes

Immunisation against Infectious Disease

8.5.5 The PPD preparation for the Mantoux test is supplied in ampoules containing 1.0ml, the contents of an ampoule being sufficient for several tests. For tests in patients in whom tuberculosis is suspected, the commercially available dilution of 10 units/ml should be used.

8.5.6 *The multiple puncture test (Heaf test)*
For this test the Heaf Multiple Puncture Apparatus (commonly known as the Heaf gun) is used. A puncture of 2mm depth is recommended for all children aged 2 years or more; under that age a puncture of 1mm is sufficient.

8.5.7 PPD for the Heaf test contains 100,000 units/ml and is supplied in packs of five ampoules of 1.0ml, each ampoule nominally being sufficient for 50 tests (depending on technique). The solution is applied to a clean dry area of the forearm with a sterile glass rod, platinum loop or needle attached to a syringe which should not be allowed to come into contact with the skin. The PPD is smoothed over by the end plate of the apparatus, which is then pressed firmly at right angles to the skin surface and the needles released. Excess PPD is then removed.

8.5.8 Results may be read any time from 3 to 10 days after puncture. A positive result should be recorded only when there is a palpable induration around at least four puncture points. Grades are defined as follows in the Heaf test:
   Grade 1   at least 4 small indurated papules
   Grade 2   an indurated ring formed by confluent papules
   Grade 3   solid induration 5 to 10mm wide
   Grade 4   induration over 10mm wide

8.5.9 It is now generally accepted that Grade 1 reactions in individuals who have not previously received BCG vaccination are usually not related to infection with Mycobacterium tuberculosis and they may therefore be offered vaccination.

8.5.10 Various estimates have been made of the correlation between the Mantoux test results and the grades of the Heaf test. As an approximation, a Heaf test response intermediate between Grade 2 and Grade 3 may be taken as equivalent to a Mantoux positive reaction following 0.1ml PPD 100 units/ml (dose of 10 units).

8.5.11 *Disinfection of the Heaf gun*

Disinfection of the Heaf gun should be carried out before each test and at the conclusion of the tuberculin testing session. The recommended method of disinfection is a three-stage process which requires an interval of two minutes or more between consecutive tests with any one instrument. Therefore at least three guns should be available for each team and they should be disinfected and used in rotation. Three guns will sustain a testing rate of 90 patients an hour with the required interval for disinfecting and cooling.

8.5.12 The three stages of the disinfection process are: immersion in spirit; burning off of the spirit; and cooling of the gun. The end of the instrument should first be immersed in 95% alcohol to a depth that totally covers the end-plate and the needles but does not wet the body of the gun. Industrial Methylated Spirit BP should be used (see footnote). Immersion should be maintained for at least 60 seconds. The gun is then withdrawn and held at an angle of 45° to the vertical with the end-plate directed upwards. The spirit is set alight by momentary contact with a flame from which the gun is removed on ignition and the spirit is allowed to burn until the flame goes out. Ensure that the needles do not become contaminated whilst cooling for which a further 30 seconds should be allowed. NEVER use a Heaf gun until you have personally supervised its disinfection in this manner.

8.5.13 An alternative to this disinfection technique involves fitting a replacement autoclaved head and needle block for each test. If a sufficient number of spare heads is available, this may prove practical.

8.5.14 Another alternative technique uses a Heaf gun with a magnetic head that holds a 6-point steel plate which is removable and separately

---

FOOTNOTE: Industrial Methylated Spirit BP should be used. This is a colourless preparation containing 95% ethyl alcohol adulterated with wood naphtha. It is virucidal and will burn readily but note that this is a volatile liquid that may create a highly flammable vapour if left in an open vessel near a naked flame. Mineralised methylated spirits (the violet preparation sold retail for general use) and Surgical Spirit BP contain only 90% alcohol plus other adulterated substances that may inhibit flammability. They are not satisfactory.

sterilisable. A recent study (8.11) has shown a high false negative rate for this technique and it has not been proved possible to recommend a method of disinfection for the magnetic head that presents fewer practical difficulties than the method described above for fixed-head guns. Use of this device is not recommended.

8.5.15 *Maintenance of the Heaf gun*

The Heaf gun should be checked carefully before use to ensure that the needles are sharp, clean and not displaced in their retaining plate. It is good practice to replace needles every six months if the gun is in regular use. Cleaning between tuberculin testing sessions can be carried out using hot detergent solution and a stiff brush but thorough rinsing in distilled water after cleaning is important. Periodical servicing of the guns by the manufacturer is recommended.

8.6 Positive reactors

8.6.1 Those with strongly positive reactions to a test for hypersensitivity to tuberculoprotein should be referred for further investigation and supervision as they may be suffering from active tuberculosis. A strongly positive reaction may be defined as a Heaf test response of Grade 3 or 4, or 15mm or more induration after a Mantoux test using 0.1ml PPD 100 units/ml.

8.7 Side effects and adverse reactions to BCG vaccine

8.7.1 Normally a local reaction develops at the site of the vaccination within 2 to 6 weeks. It begins as a small papule which slowly increases in size for 2 to 3 weeks; occasionally a shallow ulcer up to 10mm in diameter may develop. If this discharges, a temporary dry dressing may be used until a scab forms but it is essential that air should not be excluded. The lesion slowly subsides after about two months, and eventually heals leaving only a small scar. An impermeable dressing should only be applied for a very short period for example to permit swimming, as it can delay healing and result in a large scar.

8.7.2 Faulty injection technique is the most frequent cause of severe injection site reactions (large ulcers and abscesses).

8.7.3 In order to ensure that these are reduced to a minimum, it is necessary for vaccinators to be familiar with interpretation of the results of tuberculin tests and also to be skilled in the technique of intradermal injection. *The use of jet injectors is not recommended.*

8.7.4 Complications following BCG vaccination, apart from these injection site reactions, are rare and mostly consist of adenitis with or without suppuration and discharge. A minor degree of adenitis may occur in the weeks following vaccination and should not be regarded as a complication. Very rarely a lupoid type of local lesion has been reported. A very few cases characterised by widespread dissemination of the injected organisms have been reported. Anaphylactoid reactions can occur.

8.7.5 It is important that all complications should be noted and a full record kept. Serious or unusual complications (including abscess and keloid scarring) should be reported to the Committee on Safety of Medicines using the yellow card system. Every effort should be made to recover the causative organism from any lesion constituting a serious complication and have it identified. Complications following vaccination should be reported to a chest physician.

8.8 Contraindications and precautions

8.8.1 BCG vaccine should NOT be given to:
   a. Patients receiving corticosteroid or immunosuppressive treatment (including general radiation), those suffering from malignant conditions such as lymphoma, leukaemia, Hodgkin's disease or other tumours of the reticulo-endothelial system, those in whom the normal immunological mechanism may be impaired, as in hypogammaglobulinaemia and those known to be HIV positive.
   b. Although no harmful effects on the fetus have been observed from BCG vaccination during pregnancy, it is preferable to avoid vaccination in the early stages and if possible to delay until after delivery.
   c. Persons with positive sensitivity tests to tuberculo-protein. Those with Heaf Grade 1 reactions, unless previously vaccinated, may be regarded as tuberculin negative and in the absence of contraindications, offered vaccination.
   d. Persons with pyrexia.
   e. Those with generalised septic skin conditions. If eczema exists, a vaccination site should be chosen that is free from skin lesions.

8.8.2 An interval of at least 3 weeks should be allowed between the administration of BCG vaccine and any other live vaccine, whichever is given first. No further immunisation should be given for at least three months in the arm used for BCG vaccination because of the risk of regional lymphadenitis.

8.8.3 Even if performed in the few weeks after exposure to infection, before tuberculin sensitivity has developed, vaccination will do no harm. There is some advantage in delaying BCG vaccination of a tuberculin negative contact for about 6 weeks, having segregated the individual from any sputum smear-positive index case. After 6 weeks from the last known contact, the skin test should be repeated and vaccination carried out only if this test is negative. However, it is better to vaccinate without segregation than not to vaccinate at all. If in such circumstances isoniazid is to be administered prophylactically, the use of isoniazid-resistant BCG vaccine should be considered.

8.9 Record keeping and surveillance

8.9.1 It is important that individual records be available to show the vaccination state and the result of tuberculin skin testing. It is desirable that these records be completed for every person skin-tested or vaccinated under Health Authority arrangements and the records should be kept for at least 10 years.

8.9.2 BCG vaccination of hospital staff (including medical and dental students) should be recorded on an appropriate form. If staff or students move to another hospital or to another medical or dental school, the record card should be transferred.

8.10 Supply

8.10.1 In England and Wales, supplies of dried BCG vaccine (intradermal) and Tuberculin PPD are distributed to users once a month. In Scotland, the Health Boards order BCG vaccine direct from Vestric as and when required but Tuberculin PPD is distributed to users monthly. In Northern Ireland, Health and Social Services Boards order both BCG vaccine and PPD directly from Vestric.

8.10.2 Orders covering at least one month's requirement should be submitted on the user's own order form to reach the appropriate supply department by the first day of the month preceding the month when the materials are required, eg materials for use in August should be ordered by 1 July. The order should be sent to:

<table>
<tr><td>England
(BCG vaccine
(PPD</td><td>Department of Health & Social Security
Procurement Directorate
14 Russell Square
London WC1B 5EP
Tel. 01-636 6811</td></tr>
<tr><td>Scotland
(PPD only</td><td>The Central Infusion Fluids Laboratory
Knightswood Hospital
Glasgow G13 2XG
Tel. 041-954 8183</td></tr>
<tr><td>Wales
(BCG vaccine
(PPD</td><td>Welsh Office Common Services Authority
Heron House
35–43 Newport Road
Cardiff CF2 1SB
Tel. 0222 471234 extension 2068</td></tr>
</table>

8.11 Bibliography

MacHale EM and O'Shea MEB
The Heaf Test; a comparison of two types of Heaf gun
Irish Medical Journal 1987; 80; 400–1.

9 Rubella

9.1 Introduction

9.1.1 Rubella is a mild infectious disease, most common among children aged 4–9 years. It causes a transient erythematous rash, lymphadenopathy involving post-auricular and sub-occipital glands and occasionally in adults, arthritis and arthralgia. Clinical diagnosis is unreliable since the symptoms are often fleeting and can be caused by other viruses; in particular, the rash is NOT diagnostic of rubella. The incubation period is 14–21 days and the period of infectivity from 1 week before until 4 days after the onset of rash.

9.1.2 Because the rash is not diagnostic and also because infection can occur with no clinical symptoms, acute rubella can only be confirmed by laboratory tests. Diagnosis of acute infection requires either;
   i) paired sera, the first taken within 2–3 days of onset of rash and the second from 8–9 days after the onset to demonstrate appearance of rubella antibody; or
   ii) a single blood sample from 7 days after the onset of rash for estimation of rubella-specific IgM antibody; this may be detectable up to 6 weeks.

9.1.3 Maternal rubella infection in the first 8–10 weeks of pregnancy results in fetal damage in up to 90% of infants and multiple defects are common. The risk of damage declines to about 10–20% by 16 weeks; after this stage of pregnancy fetal damage is rare. Fetal defects include mental handicap, defects of vision and hearing, congenital heart disease, retardation of intra-uterine growth, and inflammatory lesions of brain, liver, lungs and bone marrow. Any combination of these defects may occur; the only defects which commonly occur alone are perceptive deafness and pigmentary retinopathy following infection after the first 8 weeks of pregnancy. Some infected infants may appear normal at birth but perceptive deafness may be detected later.

9.2 Rubella vaccine

9.2.1 The rubella virus was isolated in cell cultures in 1962. Vaccines were prepared from strains of attenuated virus and have been licensed in the UK since 1970. All rubella vaccine used in the UK contains the Wistar RA 27/3 strain grown in human diploid cells.

9.2.2 Rubella vaccine is a freeze dried preparation. It must be stored in the dried state at 2–8°C (NOT frozen) and reconstituted with the diluent fluid supplied by the manufacturer; it must be used within 1 hour of reconstitution. For both children and adults the dose is 0.5 ml given by subcutaneous injection.

9.2.3 One dose of vaccine promotes an antibody response in over 95% of vaccinees. In girls who were among the first to be vaccinated in the UK, vaccine-induced antibody has shown little decline after nearly 20 years. In countries where rubella is no longer endemic, vaccine-induced antibody has been shown to persist for over 15 years. Protection against clinical rubella appears to be long-term even in the presence of declining antibody.

9.2.4 A few recipients fail to produce antibody. It is therefore essential that any pregnant woman who is exposed to rubella should be serologically investigated, irrespective of her vaccination history (9.1.2).

9.2.5 The vaccine virus is not transmitted from vaccinees to susceptible contacts. There is thus no risk to pregnant women from contact with recently vaccinated individuals.

9.3 Recommendations (and see Section 10)

9.3.1 i. All girls between their 10th and 14th birthdays should be vaccinated against rubella. A history of rubella should be disregarded because of the unreliability of diagnosis.

ii. Non-pregnant seronegative women of child-bearing age should be vaccinated and advised not to become pregnant within 1 month of vaccination.

9.3.2 Vaccination should be avoided in early pregnancy; doctors should ascertain the date of the LMP. However despite active surveillance in USA, UK and Germany no case of congenital rubella syndrome has

Immunisation against Infectious Disease

been reported following inadvertant vaccination shortly before or during pregnancy. There is thus no evidence that the vaccine is teratogenic; termination of pregnancy following vaccination should therefore NOT be routinely recommended. The potential parents should be given this information before making a decision about termination.

9.3.3 General practitioners are uniquely placed to ensure that all women of child-bearing age have been screened for rubella antibody and vaccinated where necessary. Opportunities for screening also arise during ante-natal care, and at family planning, infertility and occupational health clinics. In such cases general practitioners must be informed of the results. Every effort must be made to identify and vaccinate sero-negative women. All women should be informed of the result of their antibody test.

9.3.4 Serological testing of non-pregnant women should be performed whenever possible before vaccination, but need not be undertaken where this might interfere with the acceptance or delivery of vaccine. Pregnancy should be avoided for 1 month.

9.3.5 Women found to be seronegative on ante-natal screening should be vaccinated after delivery and before discharge from the maternity unit. If anti-D immunoglobulin is required, the two may be given at the same time in different sites with separate syringes. While it has now been established that anti-D immunoglobulin does not interfere with the antibody response to vaccine, blood transfusion does inhibit the response in up to 50% of vaccinees. In such cases a test for antibody should be performed 8 weeks later, with revaccination if necessary. If rubella vaccine is not given post-partum before discharge, the general practitioner MUST be informed of the need for this. Alternatively it can be given at the post-natal visit. The risk of rubella infection in pregnancy is greater for parous than for nulliparous women because their own children are a source of infection; ALL WOMEN FOUND ON ANTE-NATAL SCREENING TO BE SUSCEPTIBLE TO RUBELLA SHOULD BE VACCINATED AFTER DELIVERY AND BEFORE THE NEXT PREGNANCY.

9.3.6 To avoid the risk of transmitting rubella to pregnant patients, all health service staff, both male and female, should be screened and those sero-negative vaccinated.

9.3.7 Rubella vaccine may be given to HIV positive individuals in the absence of contraindications.

9.4 Adverse reactions

9.4.1 Mild reactions such as fever, sore throat, lymphadenopathy, rash, arthralgia and arthritis may occur following vaccination. Symptoms usually begin 1–3 weeks after vaccination and are transient; joint symptoms are more common in women than in young girls. Neurological symptoms have been reported following rubella vaccination but a causal relationship has not been established.

9.4.2 Serious reactions following rubella vaccination should be reported to the Committee on Safety of Medicines using the yellow card system.

9.5 Contraindications

See Sections 1.2.2 and 1.2.3 of Introduction.

9.5.1 Rubella vaccine is a live virus vaccine and the contraindications to such vaccines should be observed;

    a. Vaccination should be postponed if the patient is suffering from a febrile illness until recovery is complete.

    b. Rubella vaccine should not be given to a woman known to be pregnant, and pregnancy should be avoided for 1 month after vaccination, but see 9.3.2.

    c. The vaccine should not be administered to patients receiving high dose corticosteroid (see 1.2.2 d) or immunosuppressive treatment including general radiation; or to those suffering from malignant conditions such as lymphoma, leukaemia, Hodgkin's disease or other tumours of the reticulo-endothelial system, or where the normal immunological mechanism may be impaired as, for example, in hypogammaglobulinaemia.

    d. If it is necessary to administer more than one live virus vaccine at the same time, they may be given simultaneously at different sites unless a combined preparation is used. If not given simultaneously they should be separated by an interval of at least 3 weeks. It is also recommended that a 3-week interval should be allowed between the administration of a live virus vaccine such as rubella vaccine and BCG.

e. Rubella vaccine should not be given within 3 months of an injection of immunoglobulin.

9.5.2 Rubella vaccines contain traces of neomycin and/or polymyxin, but this is not a contraindication except in known cases of hypersensitivity.

9.6 Surveillance

9.6.1 Any child with congenital rubella defects, or with symptoms suggestive of congenital rubella, or with laboratory evidence of intra-uterine infection without symptoms should be notified to one of the 2 Central Registries of the National Congenital Rubella Surveillance Scheme as follows:

a. Thames, Wessex, South Western, Oxford, East Anglia and Scotland:
Dr. Helen Holzel,
Department of Microbiology,
Hospital for Sick Children,
Great Ormond Street, London WC1N 3JH.
Tel. 01-405 9200. ext. 5285/6, 2417

b. West Midlands, Trent, Mersey, North Western, Northern, Yorkshire and Wales:
Professor RW Smithells,
Department of Paediatrics and Child Health,
D Floor,
The Clarendon Wing,
Leeds General Infirmary,
Belmont Grove,
Leeds LS2 9NS.
Tel. 0532 432799. ext 3909/3900

9.6.2 The two Registries are investigating the effects of rubella vaccination in pregnancy. If a woman is given rubella vaccine in pregnancy, or becomes pregnant within 1 month of vaccination, the relevant Central Registry should be notified as soon as possible. Arrangements will then be made for the appropriate clinical and virological examination of the new-born infant, and for subsequent follow-up.

9.7 Investigation of pregnant women in contact with rubella

A blood sample should be taken as soon as possible after the contact with rubella and sent to the laboratory with date of LMP and date of contact. A second sample should be taken 2 weeks later and if this is negative, a third may be requested after another two weeks.

9.8 Immunoglobulin

Post-exposure prophylaxis with immunoglobulin does not prevent infection in non-immune contacts although it may reduce the likelihood of clinical symptoms. It is not recommended for protection of pregnant women exposed to rubella (see Appendix).

9.9 Supplies

3 freeze-dried live vaccines are available, all containing the same strain, Wistar RA 27/3:

Almevax	Wellcome Foundation. Tel. 0270 583151
Ervevax	Smith Kline and French. Tel. 0707 325111
Meruvax	Morson. Tel. 0992 467272

9.9.1 Bibliography

Hanshaw J and Dudgeon JA,
'Rubella', in Viral Diseases of the fetus and new-born, 17–96.
WB Saunders, London 1978.

Consequences of confirmed maternal rubella at different stages of pregnancy.
Miller E, Cradock-Watson JE, Pollock TM
Lancet 1982, ii, 781–4.

Immunisation against Infectious Disease

Rubella vaccination: persistance of antibodies for up to 16 years.
O'Shea, S, et al
BMJ 1982, 285, 253.

Rubella vaccination and pregnancy: preliminary report of a national survey.
Shepherd S, Smithells RW, Dickson A, Holzel H
BMJ 1986, 292, 727.

National Congenital Rubella Surveillance Programme 1.7.71–30.6.84. Smithells RW, Sheppard S, Holzel H, Dickson A
BMJ 1985. 291. 40–41.

Some current issues relating to rubella vaccine.
Preblud S
JAMA 1985. 254 (2) 253–6.

Rubella susceptibility and the continuing risk of infection in pregnancy.
Miller CL, Miller E, Waight PA
BMJ 1987. 294. 1277–8.

10 Measles/Mumps/Rubella vaccine

10.1 Introduction

10.1.1 Rubella vaccine was introduced in the UK in 1970 for the vaccination of pre-pubertal girls and non-immune women. The aim of this selective policy was to protect women of child-bearing age from the risks of rubella in pregnancy. It was not intended to prevent the circulation of the rubella virus which was considered necessary to provide natural immunity and to boost vaccine-induced antibody. Selective vaccination increased the proportion of ante-natal women with rubella antibody from 85–90% before 1970 to 97–98% in 1987. However, over 2% of susceptible pregnant women still contract rubella; in 1986 and 1987, 362 infections in pregnancy were confirmed by laboratories in England and Wales. Many such pregnancies are terminated when infection is diagnosed in time. When this is not possible, Congenital Rubella Syndrome (CRS) may result, particularly in the first 9 weeks when fetal damage occurs in up to 90% of infections. On average 20 cases of CRS are still notified annually.

10.1.2 Rubella is most common among children aged 4 to 9 years who thus present a risk of infection to non-immune pregnant women, particularly their mothers. To eliminate the circulation of rubella amongst young children, the EXISTING rubella vaccination policy will be REINFORCED with the mass vaccination of young children of both sexes.

10.1.3 A combined measles/mumps/rubella vaccine (MMR) will be introduced with the aim of ELIMINATING rubella, CRS, measles and mumps. To achieve this, the target uptake for MMR vaccine for children aged 1–2 must be that already set for measles vaccine; at least 90% by 1990. In practical terms, this means every child without a valid contraindication. The target for children aged 4–5 must also be 90%; until the first cohort to receive MMR vaccine aged 1–2 years reaches school age, a high uptake of MMR must be achieved in children aged 4–5 years.

10.1.4 The mumps vaccine component will be included because of the morbidity resulting from mumps. It is the cause of about 1200 hospital admissions each year in England and Wales. In the under 15 age group it is the most common cause of viral meningitis; it can also cause permanent deafness. In the USA where mumps vaccine (as MMR) has been routinely used for over 20 years, there has been a dramatic decrease in reported cases of mumps and complications at all ages. The vaccine has been popular wherever it has been introduced and has increased the uptake of measles vaccine when the two have been combined.

10.1.5 From October 1st 1988, MMR vaccine will replace measles vaccine for all eligible children. Single antigen measles vaccine will not be given routinely after this date; single antigen rubella vaccine WILL still be used for school-girls aged 10–14 years and non-immune women (10.2.4 and 10.2.5).

10.1.6 Health Authorities will have an obligation to ensure that every child has received MMR vaccine by the time of entry to primary school, unless there is a valid contraindication, parental refusal, or laboratory evidence of previous infection. Vaccination records should be checked; where there is no record of MMR vaccination or where the child has received single antigen measles vaccine, parents will be advised that their children should receive MMR vaccine.

10.1.7 MMR vaccine can be given to children of any age whose parents request it, and also to non-immune adults. However since measles, mumps and rubella are most common before the age of entry to secondary school, mass vaccination after the age of 11 when 80–90% have already acquired antibody would have little effect on the incidence. For maximum effect, vaccine must be given soon after the 1st birthday, and at the latest before the age of 5.

10.2 Recommendations

10.2.1 *Children of both sexes aged 1–2 years*
MMR vaccine will replace measles vaccine in the second year of life, or after this age if appointments have been missed. For children whose parents refuse MMR vaccine, single antigen measles vaccine will be available.

10.2.2 *Children of both sexes aged 4–5 years before starting primary school*
MMR vaccine will be given to children whose parents consent, unless there is one of the following:
  a) A documented record of MMR vaccination.
  b) A valid contra-indication. (10.5)
  c) Laboratory evidence of immunity to measles, mumps and rubella.

MMR VACCINE SHOULD BE GIVEN IRRESPECTIVE OF PREVIOUS MEASLES VACCINE OR A HISTORY OF MEASLES, MUMPS OR RUBELLA INFECTION.

10.2.3 MMR vaccine can be given at the time of the booster dose of diphtheria/tetanus and poliomyelitis vaccines. Because the DT injection can be more painful, MMR vaccine should be injected first. The DT booster should be given with a separate syringe and needle in the opposite limb; alternatively a second appointment can be made.

10.2.4 *Rubella vaccination for girls aged 10–14 years*
This will continue unchanged with single antigen rubella vaccine and the present target of 95%. When a high uptake of MMR vaccine in young children has been achieved and maintained and the elimination of rubella has been demonstrated, the decision may be taken to stop the vaccination of schoolgirls. Vaccination of boys at this age is not proposed for reasons given in 10.1.7. There is evidence that vaccine-induced antibody is long-lasting even in the absence of endemic rubella; it is not therefore envisaged that booster injections of rubella vaccine will be necessary.

10.2.5 *Rubella vaccination of non-immune women before pregnancy and after delivery*
This will continue unchanged with single antigen rubella vaccine; every effort should be made to ensure the vaccination of all non-immune women before and after pregnancy.

10.2.6 HIV-positive individuals may be given MMR vaccine in the absence of contraindications (10.5).

10.3 MMR vaccine

This is a freeze-dried preparation supplied with separate ampoules of diluent. It should be stored in a refrigerator at 2–8°C and protected from light. It should be reconstituted with the diluent supplied by the manufacturer and used within 1 hour. The dose is 0.5 ml given by intramuscular or deep subcutaneous injection. The vaccine will be available from 2 manufacturers, Smith Kline and French (SKF) and Merieux UK; both vaccines contain the same strains of virus:

Measles;   Schwartz strain, as in Mevilin and Rimevax measles vaccine.
Rubella;   RA 27/3, as in Almevax rubella vaccine.
Mumps;   Urabe AM/9. This has been in use in the SKF vaccine in Europe and Asia for 3–4 years.

10.4 Adverse reactions

As with measles vaccine, malaise, fever and/or a rash may occur, most commonly about a week after vaccination and lasting about 2–3 days. Parotid swelling occasionally occurs, usually in the third week; children with post-vaccination symptoms are not infectious. Parents will be given information and advice for reducing fever, including the use of paracetomol in the period 5–10 days after vaccination.

10.4.1 Serious reactions should be reported to the Committee on Safety of Medicines using the yellow card system.

10.5 Contraindications

See Sections 1.2.2 and 1.2.3 of Introduction.

i) Children with untreated malignant disease or altered immunity; those receiving immunosuppressive or X-ray therapy or high-dose steroids.
ii) Children who have received another live vaccine by injection within 3 weeks.
iii) Children with allergies to neomycin or kanamycin or a history of anaphylaxis due to any cause.
iv) Children with acute febrile illness when they present for vaccination; this should be deferred.
v) If MMR vaccine is given to adult women, pregnancy should be avoided for one month, as for rubella vaccine. (9.3.2 and 9.5.1,b)

vi) MMR vaccine should not be given within 3 months of an injection of immunoglobulin.

10.5.1 Children with a personal or close family history of convulsions SHOULD be given MMR vaccine, provided the parents understand that there may be a febrile response. As for all children, advice for reducing fever will be given. IMMUNOGLOBULIN AS PREVIOUSLY USED WITH MEASLES VACCINE MUST NOT BE GIVEN WITH MMR VACCINE SINCE THE IMMUNE RESPONSE TO RUBELLA AND MUMPS MAY BE INHIBITED. Doctors should seek specialist advice rather than refuse vaccination (1.5).

10.5.2 *Allergy to egg*
This is only a contraindication if the child has had an anaphylactic reaction (generalised urticaria, swelling of the mouth and throat, difficulty in breathing, hypotension or shock) following food containing egg. Dislike of egg or refusal to eat it is NOT a contra-indication.

10.6 Post-exposure prophylaxis for measles

Either single antigen measles vaccine or MMR vaccine can be used for prophylaxis after exposure to MEASLES; to be effective it must be given within 72 hours of contact. The antibody response to the rubella and mumps components is too slow for effective prophylaxis after exposure to these infections.

10.7 Surveillance

The effect of the addition of mass MMR vaccine to selective rubella vaccination of girls and non-immune women will be monitored by the following methods:–

10.7.1 A continuing study to monitor the proportion of ante-natal women susceptible to rubella by age and parity.

10.7.2 Continued monitoring of the number and outcome of rubella infections in pregnancy, rubella terminations and notified cases of CRS.

10.7.3 Surveillance of antibody to measles, mumps and rubella by age.

Immunisation against Infectious Disease

10.7.4 Uptake of vaccine at each age by District.

10.7 Bibliography

1. Consequences of confirmed maternal rubella at different stages of pregnancy
Miller E, Cradock-Watson JE, Pollock TM
Lancet 1982, ii, 781–4.

2. Effect of selective vaccination on rubella susceptibility and infection in pregnancy
Miller CL, Miller E, Sequeira PJ, Cradock-Watson JE, Longson M, Wiseberg E
Br. Med. J 1985. 291, 1398–1401.

3. Rubella susceptibility and the continuing risk of infection in pregnancy
Miller CL, Miller E, Waight PA
Br. Med J. 1987. 294. 1277–8.

11 Influenza

11.1 Introduction

11.1.1 Influenza is an acute viral disease of the respiratory tract characterised by the abrupt onset of fever, chills, headache, myalgia and sometimes prostration. Coryza and sore throat are common and a dry cough is almost invariable. It is usually a self-limiting disease with recovery in 2–7 days. There is serological evidence of asymptomatic infection. Influenza is highly infectious, spreading rapidly in institutions. It derives its importance from the speed with which epidemics evolve and the severity of the complications, notably bacterial pneumonia. These features account for the widespread morbidity affecting all age groups, but particularly the elderly and chronic sick. Mortality, measured by the number of excess deaths attributed to "influenza", is in the region of three to four thousand even in winters when the incidence is low.

11.1.2 There are three types of influenza virus: A, B and C, the latter being of little importance. Epidemic influenza is usually caused by influenza A which attacks all age-groups, with the highest incidence in children and adolescents. Outbreaks due to Influenza A occur in most years, those due to Influenza B at intervals of several years. Influenza A viruses are antigenically labile and the principal surface antigens, the haemagglutin and neuraminidase, undergo antigenic changes. Major changes (so-called 'antigenic shifts') occur periodically and are responsible for the emergence of sub-types which may cause pandemics. More minor changes (so-called 'antigenic drifts') occur more frequently and are responsible for the interpandemic prevalence of influenza. Marked antigenic drift may be followed by large winter epidemics, but it is rarely possible to forecast the extent of outbreaks.

11.2 Influenza vaccine

11.2.1 Influenza vaccine formulation is reviewed annually and when significant alterations in antigen have occurred; changes in the composition are made to counter these 'antigenic shifts' and 'antigenic drifts'.

11.2.2 Influenza virus vaccine is inactivated and is available in 3 forms, each prepared from virus cultured in embryonated hen's eggs.

  a. 'Whole-virus' vaccine containing inactivated influenza virus purified by zonal ultra-centrifugation.
  b. 'Split virus' vaccine, a partially purified influenza vaccine containing disrupted virus particles prepared by treating whole virus particles with organic solvents or detergents and separating by zonal ultra-centrifugation.
  c. 'Surface antigen' vaccine, containing highly purified haemagglutinin and neuraminidase antigens prepared from disrupted virus particles. The antigens may be adsorbed on to aluminium hydroxide.

11.2.3 The vaccines may contain the antigens of only one strain of virus (monovalent) but more commonly are bivalent or trivalent, and contain antigens of the current influenza A and influenza B virus strains. 'Surface antigen' vaccines cause fewer adverse reactions in children than "whole-virus" vaccines, and can be used in all age groups.

11.2.4 The vaccines should be stored at 2–8°C and be protected from light. The vaccine should be allowed to reach room temperature before being given by deep subcutaneous or intramuscular injection.
  (a) A separate syringe and needle should be used for each recipient.
  (b) Multidose jet injectors should not be used.

11.2.5 Currently available influenza vaccines confer about 70 per cent protection against infection for about a year. Low levels of protection may persist for a further one to two years if the prevalent strain remains the same, or undergoes only minor 'antigenic drift'. To provide continuing protection annual immunisation is necessary with vaccine containing the most recent strains.

11.3 Recommendations

11.3.1 Recommendations to doctors on the use of influenza vaccine are issued by the Department of Health and Social Security in an annual letter from the Chief Medical Officer. The most recent statement should be consulted for details of the composition and dosage of available vaccines.

11.3.2 Vaccination is not recommended for the attempted control of the general spread of influenza. Individual protection with an appropriate inactivated vaccine should be considered for persons at special risk provided that vaccine is not contraindicated (11.5). These groups include persons, especially the elderly, suffering from the following conditions:–
  a. chronic pulmonary disease
  b. chronic heart disease
  c. chronic renal disease
  d. diabetes, and other less common endocrine disorders
  e. conditions involving immunosuppressive therapy.

11.3.3 The vaccine should be considered for elderly persons and children living in residential homes and long-stay hospitals.

11.3.4 To minimise the risk of febrile reactions after influenza vaccine in children, purified surface antigen vaccine should be used. The recommended lower age limit for vaccination of children is four years of age.

11.3.5 Vaccination of Health Service staff is indicated only for those individuals at increased risk owing to medical disorders such as those above. In the event of a pandemic or other major outbreak, advice would be given about vaccination of staff particularly liable to exposure.

11.4 Adverse reactions

11.4.1 Local reactions, consisting of redness and induration at the injection site lasting 1 to 2 days may occur in up to a third of recipients but these are usually mild. Recent influenza virus vaccines have been associated with few side-effects; two types have been described:
  a. Fever, malaise, myalgia beginning 6–12 hours after vaccination and persisting 1–2 days. This occurs more often in children than adults, and more frequently with whole virus vaccine than surface antigen vaccine.
  b. Immediate responses of an allergic nature resulting in urticaria or respiratory expressions of hypersensitivity. These are very rare.

11.4.2 Adverse reactions to influenza vaccine should be reported to the Committee on Safety of Medicines using the yellow card system.

11.5 Contraindications

See Sections 1.2.2 and 1.2.3 of Introduction.

11.5.1 a) Individuals with hypersensitivity to eggs should not be given influenza vaccine as residual egg protein is present in minute quantities. The vaccine should not be used in persons hypersensitive to polymyxin or neomycin as traces of these antibiotics may be present.

b) Pregnancy. Some evidence from past pandemic experience suggests that influenza in pregnancy is associated with increased risks of maternal mortality, and congenital malformations and leukaemia in the children. Other studies have not supported these observations, thus the significance of nfluenza during pregnancy is uncertain.

There is no evidence that influenza vaccine prepared from inactivated virus causes damage to the fetus, but as with other vaccines it should not be given during pregnancy unless there is a specific risk.

11.6 Management of outbreaks

11.6.1 As transmission of influenza virus is person-to-person via the respiratory tract, one method of limiting an outbreak is to interupt the chain of infection. Influenza has a higher mortality in the elderly and chronic sick, and contact for them with infected people should be avoided. Immunisation of contacts during an outbreak is not effective. Antiviral chemoprophylaxis, such as amantadine hydrochloride, may give protection against influenza A infection.

11.7 Supplies

Information on current vaccines is given in the latest CMO letter from the DHSS. Vaccines are available from:–
Evans, Tel. 0582 608308
Duphar, Tel. 0703 472281
Merieux UK Ltd. Tel. 0628 785291

11.8 Bibliography

Eickhoff TC
Immunisation against influenza: rationale and recommendations
J Infect Dis 1971; 123, 446–54.

Gross PA et al
A controlled double blind comparison of reactogenicity, immunogenicity and protective efficacy of whole-virus and split-product influenza vaccine in children
J Infect Dis 1977; 136, 623–632.

Hoskins TW, Davies JR, et al
Assessment of inactivated influenza A vaccine after 3 outbreaks of influenza A at Christ's Hospital
Lancet 1979; (i), 33–35.

Parkman PD, Galasso GH et al
Summary of clinical trials of influenza vaccines
J Infect Dis 1976; 134, 100–107.

Tyrell DAJ, Smith JWG
Vaccination against influenza A
Br Med Bull 1979; 35 (i), 77–85.

12 Hepatitis B

12.1 Introduction

12.1.1 Viral hepatitis B usually has an insidious onset with anorexia, vague abdominal discomfort, nausea and vomiting, sometimes arthralgia and rash, which often progresses to jaundice. Fever may be absent or mild. The severity of the disease ranges from inapparent infections, which can only be detected by liver function tests and/or the presence of serological markers of acute HBV infection (eg. HBsAg, anti-HBc), to fulminating fatal cases of acute hepatic necrosis. Among cases admitted to hospital the fatality rate is about one per cent. The average incubation period is 40–160 days but occasionally can be as long as 6–8 months.

12.1.2 The number of overt cases of hepatitis B identified in the UK appears to be low, averaging around 1000 reported cases a year. The prevalence of hepatitis B surface antigenaemia (HBsAg) is not known with certainty but is in the order of about one in 500 of the general adult population; often such individuals do not give a history of clinical hepatitis. A proportion of antigen carriers develop chronic hepatitis. Sometimes there is impairment of liver function tests; biopsy findings range from normal to active hepatitis, with or without cirrhosis. The prognosis of the liver disease in such individuals is at present uncertain, but it is known that some will develop hepatic cell carcinoma.

12.1.3 Certain occupational and other groups are known to be at increased risk of infection (see paragraph 12.3).

12.1.4 There are two types of immunisation product: a vaccine which induces an immune response, and a specific immunoglobulin which provides passive immunity and can give immediate but temporary protection after accidental inoculation or contamination with antigen-positive blood.

12.2.1 *Vaccine*
There are two types of hepatitis B vaccine, each containing 20 micrograms per ml of hepatitis B surface antigen (HBsAg) adsorbed on

aluminium hydroxide adjuvant (see dosage instructions in paragraph 12.3.8).

One vaccine is purified from human plasma by a combination of ultra-centrifugation and biochemical procedures, (H-B-Vax, Merck, Sharp and Dohme). The product is inactivated by a threefold process; each of these processes has been shown to inactivate not only hepatitis B virus, but also virus representatives of all known groups of virus which may infect humans, including HIV (the causative agent of AIDS).

The other type of vaccine contains hepatitis B surface antigen produced by yeast cells using a recombinant DNA technique, (Engerix B, Smith Kline and French).

The vaccine should be stored at 2–8°C but not frozen. *Freezing destroys the potency of the vaccine.*

12.2.2 *Supplies*
The following Hepatitis B vaccines are available:
H-B-Vax   Merck Sharp and Dohme 0992 467272
Engerix B   Smith Kline and French 0707 325111

12.2.3 The vaccine is effective in preventing infection in individuals who produce specific antibodies. Ten to fifteen per cent of those over the age of 40 do not respond; a smaller proportion of younger people are non-responsive and, overall, the vaccine is about 90% effective. Where it is thought necessary, post-vaccination screening for antibody response can best be done 2–4 months after the course of injections.

Non-responders should be considered for a booster dose but, as even then the response is likely to be poor, hepatitis B immunoglobulin (HBIG) may be necessary for protection if exposure to infection occurs (see 12.8).

Patients who are immunodeficient or on immunosuppressive therapy may respond less well than healthy individuals and may require larger doses of vaccine or an additional dose (see 12.3.9).

The duration of immunity is not precisely known but is of the order of three to five years. Advice on the need for further booster doses cannot yet be formulated, but individuals who are at high risk may wish to determine their antibody level periodically. If this falls below 10mlU/ml the need for a booster dose should be considered.

12.3 Recommendations

12.3.1 Vaccination should be considered for the groups of individuals discussed in the succeeding paragraphs under the headings "Health Care Personnel", "Patients and Family Contacts", and "Other Indications for Immunisation". It should be offered to those at highest risk as described in 12.3.5, although this list should not be regarded as exclusive.

12.3.2 Immunisation takes up to six months to confer adequate protection. This should be kept in mind when considering the need for individuals to have the vaccine. It is especially relevant in the case of new students and trainees.

NB. It is important that vaccination against hepatitis B does not encourage relaxation of good infection-control procedures. The vaccination does not prevent cross-infection with hepatitis B or protect against other blood-borne diseases such as HIV.

12.3.3 The vaccine should not be given to individuals known to be hepatitis B surface antigen (or antibody) positive, or to patients with acute hepatitis B, since in the former case it would be unnecessary and, in the latter, ineffective. Intimate contacts of individuals suffering from acute hepatitis B should be treated by passive immunisation (see 12.8) followed by active immunisation (this could be commenced simultaneously).

12.3.4 Hepatitis B vaccine may be given to HIV positive individuals; see 1.3, 12.2.3, 12.8.

Screening for antibodies prior to vaccination may be considered in a population where the antibody prevalence is expected to be high.

12.3.5 *Health care personnel*
Doctors, dentists, nurses, midwives and others, including students and trainees, who have direct contact with patients or their body fluids, or

are likely to experience frequent parenteral exposure to blood or blood-contaminated secretions and excretions.

Groups at highest risk in this category are:
1. Those health care personnel and others who are at risk because they are or may be directly involved in patient care in institutions or units for the mentally handicapped over a period of 6 months or more.
2. Those working in units treating known carriers of hepatitis B infection who are at risk because they are or may be directly involved in patient care over a period of 6 months or more.
3. Laboratory workers, mortuary technicians.
4. Health care personnel on secondment to work in areas of the world with a high prevalence of hepatitis B infection, if they are to be directly involved in patient care.

In the event of accidental inoculation with infectious material from a patient with hepatitis B, health-care workers should be offered combined active immunisation with hepatitis B vaccine and passive immunisation with hepatitis B immunoglobulin. If they have already been successfully vaccinated, they should be given a booster dose of vaccine unless they are known to have adequate protective levels of antibodies (see also 12.8).

12.3.6 *Patients and family contacts*
1. Patients on entry into institutions or units dealing with the mentally handicapped, especially where there is a known high prevalence of hepatitis B.

2. The immune response to the current hepatitis B vaccines is poorer in immunocomprised patients and those over 40. For example, only about 60 per cent of patients undergoing treatment by maintenance haemodialysis develop anti-HBs. It is suggested, therefore, that patients with chronic renal damage be immunised as soon as it appears likely that they will ultimately require treatment by maintenance haemodialysis or renal transplant.

3. The spouses or other consorts of carriers of hepatitis B if the potential vaccinee is negative for hepatitis B surface antigen or surface antibody.

Immunisation against Infectious Disease

4. Infants born to:

(a) mothers who are persistent carriers of hepatitis B surface antigen, particularly if hepatitis e antigen (HBeAg) or hepatitis B virus DNA is detectable or its antibody (anti-HBe) is not. The nature and size of the risk at birth varies from persistent carriage in 80–90 per cent of infants of HBeAg positive mothers to the less frequent occurrence of acute hepatitis B in infants of anti-HBe positive mothers.

It is most important to identify the infants at risk, and antenatal patients in high risk categories should be screened. These include:
- (i) All ethnic groups other than Caucasian, though Caucasians from Southern and Eastern Europe should also be considered.
- (ii) All those with a personal or family history of occupation suggestive of increased risk of exposure to hepatitis B virus (HBV).

(b) mothers HBsAg positive as a result of recent infection, particularly if HBeAg is detectable or anti-HBe is not.

Active/passive immunisation with vaccine and hepatitis B immunoglobulin is recommended for infants at risk. The first dose of vaccine should be given at birth or as soon as possible thereafter, and preferably within 12 hours. Hepatitis B immunoglobulin should be given at a contralateral site at the same time; arrangements should be made well in advance.

5. Whenever immediate protection is required, immunisation with the vaccine should be combined with simultaneous administration of hepatitis B immunoglobulin (HBIG) at a different site. It has been shown that passive immunisation with HBIG does not suppress an active immune response. A single dose of HBIG (usually 500 IU for adults; 200 IU for the newborn) is sufficient for healthy individuals. If infection has already occurred at the time of the first immunisation, virus multiplication is unlikely to be inhibited completely, but severe illness and, most importantly, the development of the carrier state of HBV may be prevented in many individuals, particularly in infants born to carrier mothers.

12.3.7 *Other indications for immunisation*

Consideration should also be given to members of the following groups, and it should be noted here that if the recommended precautions to protect against HIV infection were taken, the risk of spread of HBV would be considerably reduced.

1. *Police and Emergency Services*

The statistics of the incidence of hepatitis B do not show that, in general, members of the police, ambulance, rescue services and staff of custodial institutions are at greater risk than the general population. Nevertheless, there may be individuals within these occupations who are at higher risk and who should be considered for vaccination. Such a selection has to be decided locally by the occupational health services, or following other medical advice as appropriate.

2. *Travellers*

Those going to work in areas of the world where hepatitis B is endemic and who may be involved in the care of patients. Travellers who are likely to be in such endemic areas for a lengthy period could also be considered for vaccination because of the risk of acquiring infection from medical procedures carried out with inadequately sterilised equipment, eg. syringes and needles.

3. Morticians and embalmers.

4. Individuals who frequently change sexual partners, particularly those who are prostitutes or male homosexuals.

5. Inmates of long-term custodial institutions.

6. Parenteral drug misusers.

12.3.8 *Recommended dosage for primary immunisation*

The basic immunisation regimen consists of three doses of vaccine, with the first dose at the elected date, the second dose one month later and the third dose at six months after the first dose.

The recombinant vaccine has also been used where more rapid immunisation is required, for example with travellers when the third dose may be given at 2 months after the initial dose with a booster dose at twelve months.

Immunisation against Infectious Disease

The vaccine should normally be given intramuscularly. The injection should be given in the deltoid region, though the anterolateral thigh is the preferred site for infants. The buttock should not be used because vaccine efficacy may be reduced.

It may be given intradermally in adults and children over 10 years of age under circumstances where the skilled procedure of intradermal injection can be assured, and where post-immunisation antibody testing can be done to confirm that a satisfactory immune response has resulted.

In patients with haemophilia, the intradermal or subcutaneous route may be considered.

Doctors are however advised that until such time as the manufacturers apply for and are granted variations to their product licences for the intradermal route of administration, the use of this route would be on their own personal responsibility.

12.3.9 *Dosage schedule*
The dose is the same for each of the 3 injections.

Newborn infants and children under 10 years:
    0.5 ml intramuscularly (10 micrograms)
(For new born infants see also 12.3.6, 4.)

Adults and children over 10 years:
    1.0ml intramuscularly (20 micrograms)
    0.1ml intradermally (2 micrograms)

Immunocompromised and dialysis patients:
    2.0ml intramuscularly (40 micrograms), given as two 1.0ml doses at different sites

Alternative regime for immunocompromised patients:
    1.0ml (20 micrograms) as initial dose, repeated 1 and 2 months later, and 2ml (40 micrograms) at 6 months.

NOTE. The dosage for recombinant vaccine, Engerix B (Smith, Kline and French) is not yet established in neonates and children under 3 years. Dosage for children over 3 years is the same as for adults. The manufacturer's latest data sheet must be consulted.

12.4 Adverse reactions

Adverse reactions to hepatitis B vaccine observed to date have been generally limited to soreness and redness at the injection site if given intramuscularly.

Injection intradermally may produce a persisting nodule at the site of the injection, sometimes with local pigmentation changes.

12.4.1 It is important that adverse reactions should be reported to the Committee on Safety of Medicines by the yellow card system.

12.5 Pregnancy

Hepatitis B infection in pregnant women may result in severe disease for the mother and chronic infection of the newborn. Vaccination should not be withheld from a pregnant woman if she is in a high risk category.

12.6 Effect of vaccination on carriers

The vaccine produces neither therapeutic nor adverse effects on carriers of hepatitis B.

12.7 Contraindications

Vaccination should be postponed in individuals suffering from serious infection.

12.8 Hepatitis B immunoglobulin (HBIG). See Appendix 19.3.2

12.8.1 A specific immunoglobulin is available for passive protection against hepatitis B. It is used in the following circumstances:

Hepatitis B

a. Persons who are accidentally inoculated or who contaminate the eye or mouth or fresh cuts or abrasions of skin with blood from a known HBsAg positive person. Individuals who sustain such accidents should wash the affected area well and seek medical advice. Advice about prophylaxis after such accidents should be obtained by telephone from the nearest Public Health Laboratory. Advice following accidental exposure may also be obtained from the Hospital Control of Infection Officer or the Occupational Health Services.

b. Children born to mothers who develop acute hepatitis B in the last trimester of pregnancy or who are highly infective HBsAg carriers should be immunised in the neonatal period, beginning as soon as possible after birth, preferably within 12 hours (see paragraph 12.3,4,6 above) and not later than 48 hours.

c. Sexual consorts, (and in some circumstances a family contact judged to be at high risk) of individuals suffering from acute hepatitis B, and who are seen within one week of onset of jaundice in the contact.

12.8.2 There is no epidemiological evidence associating the administration of intramuscular immunoglobulin, either normal or specific, with seroconversion for antibodies to HIV. Not only does the processing of the plasma from which these immunoglobulins are prepared render them safe, but the screening of blood donations is now routine practice.

12.8.3 *Supplies*
Public Health Laboratory Service, either from the Central Public Health Laboratory (Tel: 01-200 6868) or via local Public Health Laboratories. Hepatitis B immunoglobulin is held in Scotland by the Blood Transfusion Service:

    Aberdeen   (0224) 681818
    Dundee   (0382) 645166
    Edinburgh   (031) 2297291
    Glasgow   (0698) 373315
    Inverness   (0463) 234151

Hepatitis B immunoglobulin is held in Northern Ireland by the Regional Virus Laboratory, Royal Victoria Hospital, Belfast. Tel: (0232) 240503.

Note: Supplies of this product are limited and demands should be restricted to patients in whom there is a clear indication for its use.

12.9 Hepatitis A

12.9.1 Hepatitis A is usually transmitted by the faecal oral route generally after the ingestion of contaminated food or drink. The disease is usually milder than hepatitis B and is very seldom fatal. A chronic carrier state is unknown and chronic liver damage is extremely unlikely. The incubation period is about 15–40 days. Outbreaks occasionally occur in this country although most cases are sporadic. Persons travelling to developing countries may be at greater risk of contracting hepatitis A.

12.9.2 Human normal immunoglobulin (HNIG) (see Appendix) offers protection against infection with hepatitis A and is normally used under the following circumstancs:
   a. to control outbreaks of hepatitis A in households and in institutions.
   b. for persons travelling to areas of poor sanitation.

12.9.3 Human normal immunoglobulin may interfere with the development of active immunity from live virus vaccines. It is, therefore, wise to administer live virus vaccines at least three weeks before the administration of immunoglobulin. If immunoglobulin has been administered first, then an interval of three months should be observed before administering a live virus vaccine.

12.9.4. *Supplies*
The Public Health Laboratory Service; in Scotland, the Blood Transfusion Service. (see 12.8.3)

13 Rabies

13.1 Introduction

13.1.1 Rabies is an acute viral infection resulting in encephalomyelitis. The onset is insidious. Early symptoms may include paraesthesiae around the site of the wound, fever, headache and malaise. The disease may present in one of two ways; hydrophobia, hallucinations, and maniacal behaviour progressing to paralysis and coma, or an ascending flaccid paralysis and sensory disturbance. Rabies is almost always fatal, with death resulting from respiratory paralysis. The incubation period is generally 2–8 weeks, but may range from 9 days to two years.

13.1.2 Infection is usually via the bite of a rabid animal, but transmission of the virus can also occur through mucous membranes, though not through intact skin. Person-to-person spread of the disease is extremely rare, but instances of transmission by corneal graft have been reported. No indigenous human rabies has been reported in the United Kingdom since 1902 although cases occur in persons infected abroad. The disease occurs in all continents except Australasia and Antarctica. Rabies in animals has spread throughout a great part of Central and Western Europe since 1945 and continues to advance westwards. In Europe foxes are predominantly infected but many other animals become infected including dogs and cats, cattle, horses, badgers, martens and deer. The prevention of rabies spreading to the UK depends on the control of imported animals. Individuals at high risk of exposure, such as animal handlers, should be given pre-exposure vaccine (see 13.3.1). Rabies vaccine is used for pre-exposure protection, whilst both vaccine and rabies specific immunoglobulin may be needed for rabies post-exposure treatment.

13.2 Vaccine

13.2.1 The vaccine currently available is a human diploid cell vaccine (HDCV). It is a freeze dried suspension of Wistar rabies virus strain PM/WI 38 1503-3M cultured on human diploid cells and inactivated by beta-propiolactone. For post-exposure treatment the potency of the reconstituted vaccine should be not less than $2.5 \times$ the International

Standard per 1ml dose. The freeze-dried vaccine should be stored at 4°C and used immediately after reconstitution with the diluent supplied. It may be given by deep subcutaneous, intramuscular or intradermal injection; post-vaccination antibody may not be apparent until the tenth day of a course. The antibody response may be poor if the gluteal region is used for injection.

13.2.2 Rabies-specific immunoglobulin

Passive immunisation with human rabies immunoglobulin (HRIG) provides rapid immune protection for a short period and can be used in combination with HDCV in post-exposure treatment to cover the delay associated with active immunisation. HRIG is obtained from the plasma of vaccinated human donors.

13.3 Recommendations

13.3.1 HDCV may be used for pre-exposure prophylaxis and post-exposure treatment (see under Management of Cases). Pre-exposure vaccination should be offered to those employed in the following categories:–

    a. at animal quarantine premises for imported animals and zoological establishments

    b. as carrying agents authorised to carry imported animals

    c. at approved research and acclimatisation centres where primates and other imported animals are housed

    d. at national ports of entry where contact with imported animals is likely (eg. Customs and Excise Officers)

    e. as veterinary and technical staff of the Ministry of Agriculture, Fisheries and Food (MAFF) and Department of Agriculture and Fisheries for Scotland (DAFS)

    f. as inspectors appointed by local authorities under the Diseases of Animals Act, or employed otherwise who, by reason of their employment, encounter increased risk

    g. in laboratories handling rabies virus

    h. as health workers who come into close contact with a patient with rabies

    i. as workers in enzootic areas where they may be at special risk (eg. veterinary staff or persons working in remote areas in developing countries).

All such persons at occupational risk at home and abroad are entitled to rabies vaccine free from the NHS.

Rabies vaccine is NOT recommended as a routine prophylactic measure for travellers abroad and is not available free from the NHS under these circumstances. Travellers who wish to do so can obtain vaccine on payment.

13.3.2 For pre-exposure protection, two doses of vaccine each of 1.0ml should be given four weeks apart by deep subcutaneous or intramuscular injection. A reinforcing dose is given after 12 months. Additional reinforcing doses are given every one to three years depending on the risk of exposure, and also following exposure to possible rabies. When more than one person is to be vaccinated the vaccine may be administered in smaller doses (0.1ml) by the intradermal route with the same time intervals as above. It is emphasised that intradermal vaccination is reliable only if the whole of the 0.1ml dose is properly given into the dermis. Those not experienced in intradermal technique should give a full dose by intramuscular injection. Staff who are engaged in the care of a patient with rabies may be rapidly immunised by receiving 0.1ml of vaccine intradermally in each limb (0.4ml in all) on the first day of exposure to the patient.

13.3.3 Many authorities recommend that a serological test should be carried out on all people receiving rabies vaccine for pre-exposure immunisation, to ensure that they are adequately protected.

13.4 Adverse reactions

13.4.1 HDCV may cause local reactions such as redness, swelling or pain at the site of injection within 24–48 hours of administration. Systemic reactions such as headache, fever, muscle aches, vomiting, and urticarial rashes have been reported within 24 hours. Anaphylactic shock has been reported from the USA and Guillain-Barré syndrome from Norway.

13.4.2 Suspected adverse reactions should be reported to the Committee on Safety of Medicines using the yellow card system.

13.5 Contraindications

13.5.1 There are no specific contraindications to HDCV, although if there were evidence of hypersensitivity to the first dose, subsequent doses should not be given.

13.5.2 Pre-exposure vaccine should only be given to pregnant women if the risk of exposure to rabies is high.

13.6 Management of cases

13.6.1 Should an outbreak in animals occur and a rabies-infected area be declared, vaccination would need to be offered, as appropriate, to those persons directly involved in control measures, and to veterinary surgeons and their ancillary staff working within the infected area.

13.6.2 Human rabies is a notifiable disease. In the event of a case of human rabies, the Medical Officer for Environmental Health (in Scotland the Chief Administrative Medical Officer) should be informed. Detailed advice on the management of an outbreak appears in the "Memorandum on Rabies" issued by the DHSS and SHHD in 1977.

13.6.3 Treatment should be started as soon as possible:
i) Thorough cleansing of the wound by scrubbing with soap and water under a running tap for 5 minutes.
ii) Active and, if indicated, passive immunisation.

13.6.4 1.0ml of HDCV should be given by deep subcutaneous or intramuscular injection on days 0, 3, 7, 14, 30 and 90. (Day 0 is the day the patient receives the first dose.)

13.6.5 HRIG should be given immediately. The recommended dose is 20 IU/Kg body weight, half of which should be thoroughly infiltrated into the area of the wound and the rest given intramuscularly. Local pain and low grade fever may follow the administration of HRIG, but no serious adverse reactions have been reported.

13.6.6 WHO recommendations for treatment are given in the WHO Expert Committee Report (See 13.8).

Immunisation against Infectious Disease

13.6.7 For travellers returning to this country (see 13.1.2) who report an exposure to an animal abroad treatment should be started while enquiries are made about the prevalence of rabies in the country concerned, and where possible, the condition of the biting animal. Information should be sought from PHLS Communicable Disease Surveillance Centre, London (01-200 6868); in Scotland, the Communicable Diseases (Scotland) Unit (041-946 7120); in Northern Ireland, DHSS (0232 650111).

13.6.8 For a fully vaccinated person shown to have developed antibody, a modified course of post-exposure vaccine may be given following a bite by a possibly rabid animal. Advice should be obtained from the Virus Reference Laboratory, Central Public Health Laboratory, Colindale, London (01-200 6868).

13.7 Supplies

13.7.1 a. Human diploid cell vaccine (HDCV) is manufactured by Institut Merieux, France, and is available from Merieux UK Tel. 0628 785291.

HDCV for persons in categories 13.3.1 is supplied by the DHSS and available from the PHLS Virus Reference Laboratory, Tel 01 200 6868. For persons not in these categories for whom it is not available on NHS prescription it should be obtained from commercial sources: Merieux UK Limited. (Tel. 0628 785291).

b. For post-exposure use, emergency supplies are also held in several other centres. Information may be obtained from Virus Reference Laboratory, Tel. 01 200 6868 (see 13.6.8).

c. Human rabies immunoglobulin (HRIG) is manufactured by Blood Products Laboratory and supplied through some Public Health Laboratories (see b. above).

d. Supply Centres in Scotland for HDCV and HRIG are listed in the SHHD Memorandum on Rabies.

13.8 Bibliography

WHO Expert Committee on Rabies, 7th report
Technical Report Series, 709 WHO, Geneva 1984.

14 Cholera

14.1 Introduction

14.1.1 Cholera is an acute intestinal disease caused by an enterotoxin produced by *Vibrio cholerae*, Serogroup 01, of the classical and El Tor biotypes. Cholera is characterised by sudden onset of profuse watery stools, occasional vomiting, rapid dehydration, metabolic acidosis and circulatory collapse. Over 50% of the most severe cases if untreated may die within a few hours of onset; if treated correctly, mortality is less than 1%. Mild cases with only moderate diarrhoea may occur. Asymptomatic infections are many times more frequent than those with symptoms especially with El Tor cholera. The incubation period is between 2 and 5 days but may be only a few hours.

14.1.2 The last indigenous case of cholera was reported in 1893. Between 1970 and 1987, 51 imported cases of cholera with 2 deaths were reported in England and Wales. Further importation is likely, but the risk of an outbreak is very small in any country with modern sanitation and water supplies, and high standards of food hygiene.

14.1.3 Infection is acquired from contaminated water, shellfish or other food. Even in endemic areas the risk to tourists is very small.

14.1.4 Cholera vaccine is of limited use. In endemic areas, the vaccine has been shown to reduce the incidence of overt disease by only 50%; it also fails to prevent people becoming asymptomatic carriers. Whilst the World Health Organisation (WHO) no longer recommends cholera vaccination for travel to or from cholera-infected areas, some countries still require evidence of vaccination 6 days to 6 months before entry. It is for this reason, and the fact that vaccination may confer some personal protection, that cholera vaccine is available.

14.2 Vaccine

14.2.1 Cholera vaccine consists of a heat-killed, phenol-preserved mixed suspension of the Inaba and Ogawa serotypes of *Vibrio cholerae*, serovar 01. The vaccine is effective against both the classical and the El

Immunisation against Infectious Disease 85

Tor biotypes. The protection conferred persists for 3 to 6 months, but is minimal a year after the last dose.

14.2.2 The vaccine should be stored at 2–8°C. It has a tendency, on standing, to settle out in a gelatinous form. Vigorous shaking will yield a homogeneous suspension suitable for injection. Any partly used multi-dose containers should be discarded at the end of the vaccination session.

14.3 Recommendations

14.3.1 *Cholera vaccine is indicated for the following:*
  a. People travelling to countries which require evidence of cholera vaccination. Travellers should enquire from the relevant Embassy or High Commissioner's office for current requirements. An international certificate of vaccination is no longer required by international regulations but some countries require a medical certificate. This is valid for 6 months beginning 6 days after vaccination, or the date of re-vaccination.
  b. People travelling to countries or areas where cholera is endemic or epidemic, especially if they will be living in unhygienic conditions.

14.3.2 Cholera vaccine is not indicated in the control of the spread of infection or in the management of contacts of imported cases.

14.3.3 Because of the low vaccine efficacy, vaccinees should be told that the best protection against cholera, as well as against other enteric diseases is to avoid food and water which might be contaminated.

14.3.4 A single dose of vaccine may be sufficient to satisfy the regulations of those countries still requiring proof of cholera vaccination for entry. Cholera vaccine is not recommended for children under one year of age.

14.3.5 Cholera vaccine may be given to HIV positive individuals.

14.3.6 Primary immunisation consists of two doses of vaccine given by deep subcutaneous or intramuscular injection, separated by a period of at least one week and preferably one month. Booster doses are recommended every 6 months to maintain immunity. When more than

6 months have elapsed since the last dose, a single dose is insufficient to boost immunity.

14.3.7 The recommended doses for primary and booster immunisations are:

Deep subcutaneous or intramuscular injection

Age	First dose	All subsequent doses
1–5 years	0.1ml	0.3ml
5–10 years	0.3ml	0.5ml
Over 10 years	0.5ml	1.0ml

14.4 Adverse reactions

14.4.1 Cholera vaccination will occasionally cause some local tenderness and redness at the injection site lasting 1–2 days. This may be accompanied by fever, malaise and headache. Serious reactions are rare.

14.4.2 Serious reactions should be reported to the Committee on Safety of Medicines using the yellow card system.

14.5 Contraindications

14.5.1   i) The vaccine should not be given to anyone suffering from febrile illness.

ii) Although there is no information to suggest that cholera vaccine is unsafe during pregnancy, it should only be given when this is unavoidable, ie required for travel.

iii) Repeated vaccinations may result in the development of hypersensitivity.

iv) A severe reaction to cholera vaccination is a contraindication to further doses.

14.6 Management of outbreaks

14.6.1 Cholera vaccine has no role in the management of contacts of cases, or in controlling the spread of infection. Sources of infection should be identified and appropriate measures taken. Contacts should maintain high standards of personal hygiene to avoid becoming infected. Control of the disease is based on public health measures rather than vaccination.

14.7 Supplies

14.7.1 Vials of 1.5ml and 10ml are available from the Wellcome Foundation Ltd. Tel: Crewe (0270) 583151.

14.8 Bibliography

Burgasov PN et al
Comparative study of reactions and serological response to cholera vaccines in a controlled field trial conducted in the USSR
Bull. WHO 1976; 54(2); 163–170.

Phillipines Cholera Committee
A controlled field trial of the effectiveness of intradermal and subcutaneous administration of cholera vaccine
Bull. WHO 1973; 49, 389–394.

Sommer A, Khan M, Mosley WH
Efficacy of vaccination of family contacts of cholera cases
Lancet 1973; (i), 1230–1232.

15 Typhoid

15.1 Introduction

15.1.1 Typhoid and paratyphoid fevers are systemic infections caused by bacteria of the Salmonella genus. This genus comprises almost 2000 serotypes, most of which rarely give rise to systemic invasion and usually cause only gastro-enteritis or 'food poisoning'. However, *S. typhi*, *S. paratyphi* A, B and C and occasionally other salmonella species may produce systemic infection with prolonged pyrexia, prostration and the characteristic clinical picture of 'enteric' fever. The incubation period, which depends on the size of the infecting dose, is usually one to three weeks. Whilst all cases of typhoid and paratyphoid discharge bacilli during their illness, about 10 per cent of typhoid cases continue to excrete for three months and 2 to 5% become permanent carriers; the likelihood of becoming a chronic carrier increases with age, especially in females.

15.1.2 Salmonella typhi is transmitted mainly by food and drink that has been contaminated with excreta of a human case or carrier. Recent examples of sources of outbreaks include canned corned beef (Aberdeen 1964), water supplies (Zermatt 1963) and shellfish contaminated by infected water or sewage. Typhoid is now predominantly a disease of countries where water or food supplies are liable to faecal contamination. In 1938 there were nearly 1000 notifications and 144 deaths in England and Wales attributable to typhoid but since 1960 the annual incidence has remained between about 100 and 200 notified cases. Over 80% of the cases acquire infection abroad, principally in the Indian sub-continent.

15.1.3 Combined typhoid and parathyphoid A and B vaccine is no longer available; there is thus no vaccine against paratyphoid fever.

15.2 Vaccine

15.2.1 The monovalent vaccine contains heat-killed, phenol-preserved *S. typhi* organisms at a concentration of not less than 1000 million/ml. One injection gives around 70–80% protection which fades after 1 year.

Two doses at an interval of 4–6 weeks give protection for 3 years or more. Vaccine efficacy is related to the size of the infecting dose encountered after vaccination.

15.2.2 The vaccine should be stored at 2–8°C. Any partly used multi-dose containers should be discarded at the end of the vaccination session.

15.2.3 Typhoid vaccine may be given by deep subcutaneous or intramuscular injection.

15.3 Recommendations

15.3.1 Routine typhoid vaccination is not recommended. It is advised for;
Laboratory workers handling specimens which may contain typhoid organisms.

It should be considered for;
All persons travelling abroad, with the exception of those going to Canada, USA, Australia, New Zealand and Northern Europe.

It is not recommended for contacts of a known typhoid carrier.

15.3.2 The basic course of vaccination consists of two doses separated by 4–6 weeks. (The Ministry of Defence advise a third dose after 6 months.)

   a. Adults and children over 10 years
      Deep subcutaneous/intramuscular injection
      Basic 1   0.5ml
            2   0.5ml
      Reinforcement 0.5ml (every 3 years)

   b. Children 1 to 10 years
      Deep subcutaneous/intramuscular injection
      Basic 1   0.25ml
            2   0.25ml
      Reinforcement 0.25ml (every 3 years)

15.3.3 Although two doses of vaccine are recommended, one dose is effective for a short period. Typhoid vaccine is not recommended for infants under one year as the risk of infection in infants is low. Under conditions of continued or repeated exposure to infection, a reinforcing dose of vaccine should be given every three years.

15.3.4 Typhoid vaccine may be given to HIV positive individuals in the absence of contraindications.

15.4 Adverse reactions

15.4.1 Typhoid vaccine commonly produces local reactions such as redness, swelling, pain and tenderness which may appear after two or three hours and persist for a few days. Systemic reactions include malaise, nausea, headache or pyrexia, which usually disappear within 36 hours. Neurological complications have been described but are rare. Reactions are especially common after repeated injections of typhoid vaccine, and are often more marked in persons over 35 years.

15.4.2 Severe reactions should be reported to the Committee on Safety of Medicines using the yellow card system.

15.5 Contraindications

15.5.1 a. Vaccination of children under 1 year of age is not advised because of the risk of adverse reactions, the relatively low incidence of typhoid in this age group and the relatively mild course of the disease in infants.
    b. Typhoid vaccine should not be given to subjects with acute febrile illness.
    c. Typhoid vaccine is not recommended during an outbreak of typhoid fever in the UK as no immediate protection is afforded by the vaccine. There is also some possibility of temporarily increasing susceptibility to infection. Moreover the vaccine renders the diagnosis of suspected illness more difficult because of interference with serological tests.
    d. Repeated injections of typhoid vaccine increase the risk of hypersensitivity. Re-vaccination of fully immunised adults should only

be required for those travelling to or staying in endemic areas under conditions of poor hygiene.

e. Although there is no information to suggest that typhoid vaccine is unsafe during pregnancy, it should only be used if clear indication exists.

15.6 Management of outbreaks

15.6.1 It is important that the Medical Officer for Environmental Health (MOEH) or, in Scotland, the Chief Administrative Medical Officer (CAMO) should be informed immediately whenever a patient is suspected of suffering from typhoid without waiting for laboratory confirmation.

15.6.2 Early identification of the source of infection is vital in containing this disease. Household contacts of cases, (that is, those exposed to faeces or vomit of a case, or to the same source), should be excluded from work if they are involved in food handling, until at least two, and in some cases three, negative faecal cultures have been obtained. The need for strict personal hygiene should be stressed.

15.7 Supplies

15.7.1 Vials of 1.5ml are available from the Wellcome Foundation Limited. Tel: Crewe (0270) 583151.

15.8 Bibliography

Ashcroft MT et al
A seven year field trial of two typhoid vaccines in Guyana
Lancet 1967: (ii), 1056–1059.

Cvjetanovic B, Uemara K
The present status of field and laboratory studies of typhoid and paratyphoid vaccines
Bull. WHO 1965: 32, 29–36

Galbraith NS, Barrett NJ, Sockett PN
The changing pattern of foodborne disease in England and Wales
Pub. Hlth 1987. 101; 319–328

Hejfec LB
Duration of post vaccination anti-typhoid immunity according to the results of strictly controlled field trials
J. Hyg. Epid. Microbiol. Imm. 1969: 13, 154–165.

Iwarson S, Larrson P
Intradermal versus subcutaneous immunisation with typhoid vaccine
J. Hyg. Camb. (1980): 84, 11–16.

16 Anthrax

16.1 Anthrax is an acute bacterial disease affecting the skin and, rarely, the lungs or gastro-intestinal tract. It is caused by a spore-bearing aerobic bacillus, *Bacillus anthracis* and is primarily a disease of herbivorous animals. In the UK it is rare – 9 cases notified in the last 10 years – and only affects workers exposed to infected hides, wool, hair, bristle, bone, bone meal, feeding stuffs and carcases. Spores may survive for many years, and new areas of infection may develop through the use of infected animal feed. Prevention depends on controlling anthrax in livestock and by disinfecting imported animal products. Processing of hides, wool and bone by tanning, dyeing, carbonising or acid treatment ensures that the final product carries no risk of infection. Bonemeal used as horticultural fertiliser may rarely contain anthrax spores; those handling it in bulk should wear impervious gloves which should be destroyed after use.

16.2 Vaccine

Human anthrax vaccine is the alum precipitate of the antigen found in the sterile filtrate of the Sterne strain cultures of *Bacillus anthracis*, with thiomersal preservative. It must be kept at 2–8°C and should be well shaken before being given by intramuscular injection.

16.3 Recommendations

16.3.1 Vaccination against anthrax is recommended only for workers at risk of exposure to the disease (16.1). Four injections of 0.5ml should be given, with intervals of 3 weeks between the first 3 injections and 6 months between the third and fourth. Annual reinforcing doses of 0.5ml are advised.

16.3.2 Workers at special risk should wear protective clothing. Adequate washing facilities, ventilation and dust control in hazardous industries should be provided. Prompt reporting and scrupulous medical care of skin abrasions are essential.

16.4 Adverse reactions

16.4.1 These are rare. Mild erythema and swelling lasting up to 2 days may occur at the site of the injection. Occasionally regional lymphadenopathy, mild fever and urticaria may develop.

16.4.2 Severe reactions should be reported to the Committee on Safety of Medicines using the yellow card system.

16.5 Contraindications

There are no specific contraindications. A local or general reaction to the first injection does not necessarily indicate a predisposition to reactions following subsequent injections.

16.6 Management of outbreaks

16.6.1 All cases of anthrax should be notified; an attempt should be made to confirm the diagnosis bacteriologically and the source of infection should be investigated. Penicillin is the treatment of choice. Skin lesions should be covered; any discharge or soiled articles should be disinfected. Anthrax vaccine has no role in the management of a case or outbreak.

16.7 Supplies

Anthrax vaccine is available from:
Public Health Laboratory Service;
   Communicable Disease Surveillance Centre, Tel. 01 200 6868
   Centre for Applied Microbiology and Research, Tel. 0980 610391
   Cardiff, Tel. 0222 755944
   Leeds, Tel. 0532 645011
   Liverpool, Tel. 051 525 2323

Scotland: Bridge of Earn, Tel. 073 881 2331
           Law, Tel. 0698 351100
           Peel, Tel 0896 57911

16.8 Bibliography

Editorial
Vaccine against anthrax
BMJ 1965: ii; 717–8

James DG
The epidemiology of anthrax
J Antimicrob. Chemother. 1976; 2(4); 319–20

Turnbull PC
Thoroughly modern anthrax
Abstracts of Hygiene, Bureau Hyg & Trop. Dis. 1986; 61(9);

17 Smallpox

17.1 In December 1979 the Global Commission for the Certification of Smallpox Eradication declared the world free of smallpox and this declaration was ratified by the World Health Assembly in May 1980.

THERE IS THUS NO INDICATION FOR SMALLPOX VACCINATION FOR ANY INDIVIDUAL WITH THE POSSIBLE EXCEPTION OF SOME LABORATORY STAFF AND SPECIFIC WORKERS AT IDENTIFIABLE RISK (17.2)

17.2 Recommendations

Workers in laboratories where pox viruses (such as vaccinia) are handled, and others whose work involves an identifiable risk of exposure to a pox virus, should be advised of the risk and possible need for vaccination. Advice on the need for vaccination and contraindications should be obtained from Public Health Laboratory Service Virus Reference Laboratory Tel 01 200 4400; if vaccination is considered desirable, vaccine can be obtained through PHLS on this number. Antivaccinia immunoglobulin is available from the Virus Reference Laboratory who should be consulted about its use.

18 Yellow fever

18.1 Introduction

18.1.1 Yellow fever is an acute viral infection occurring in tropical Africa and S. America; it has never been seen in Asia. It ranges in severity from non-specific symptoms to an illness of sudden onset with fever, vomiting and prostration which may progress to haemorrhage and jaundice. In indigenous populations in endemic areas fatality is about 5%; in non-indigenous individuals and during epidemics fatality may reach 50%. Two epidemiological forms, urban and jungle, are recognised although they are clinically and aetiologically identical. Only a few outbreaks of urban yellow fever have occurred in recent years. The incubation period is 2–5 days.

18.1.2 Urban yellow fever is spread from infected to susceptible persons by *Aedes aegypti*, a mosquito which lives and breeds in close association with man. Jungle yellow fever is a zoonosis transmitted among non-human hosts (mainly monkeys) by forest mosquitoes which may also bite and infect humans. These may, if subsequently bitten by *Aedes aegypti* become the source of outbreaks of the urban form of the disease.

18.1.3 Preventative measures against urban yellow fever include eradication of Aedes mosquitoes, protection from mosquitoes, and vaccination. Jungle fever can only be prevented by vaccination.

18.2 Vaccine

18.2.1 Yellow fever vaccine is a live attenuated freeze-dried preparation of the 17D strain of yellow fever virus. Each 0.5ml dose contains not less than 1000 mouse LD50 units. It is propagated in leucosis-free chick embryos and contains no more than 2 IU of neomycin and 5 IU of polymyxin per dose.

18.2.2 It should be stored at 2–8°C and protected from light. The diluent supplied for use with the vaccine should be stored below 15°C but not frozen. The vaccine should be given by deep subcutaneous injection within 1 hour of reconstitution.

18.2.3 A single dose correctly given confers immunity in nearly 100% of recipients; immunity persists for at least 10 years and may be for life.

18.3 Recommendations

18.3.1 The following should be vaccinated;
 a. Laboratory workers handling infected material.
 b. Persons aged 9 months and over travelling through or living in infected areas.

Note. A valid International Certificate of Vaccination is compulsory for entry or travel through endemic areas and may be required for those entering yellow fever receptive areas from an endemic area. Requirements should be checked with the leaflet 'The Traveller's Guide to Health – Before You Go' SA 40 or the relevant Embassy.

18.3.2 The dose is 0.5ml irrespective of age. The International Certificate is valid for 10 years from the 10th day after primary vaccination and immediately after revaccination. For travellers, yellow fever vaccine is only given at centres approved by WHO (see 18.9).

18.3.3 Revaccination every 10 years is recommended for travellers to infected areas and laboratory workers at special risk.

18.3.4 Normal human immunoglobulin obtained in the UK is unlikely to contain antibody to the yellow fever virus; the vaccine can therefore be given at the same time as an injection of immunoglobulin for travellers abroad.

18.4 Adverse reactions

18.4.1 Severe reactions are extremely rare. Five to ten per cent of recipients have mild headache, myalgia, low-grade fever or soreness at the injection site 5–10 days after vaccination.

18.4.2 The only serious reaction following 17D tissue culture vaccine has been the rare occurrence of encephalitis in young infants, all of whom have recovered without sequelae. Vaccination under 9 months is not recommended if exposure to the risk of infection can be avoided.

18.4.3 Severe reactions should be reported to the Committee on Safety of Medicines using the yellow card system.

18.5 Contraindications

18.5.1 The usual contraindications to a live virus vaccine should be observed (see 1.2.2):
i. Persons suffering from febrile illness.
ii. Patients receiving high-dose corticosteroid or immuno suppressive treatment, including radiation.
iii. Patients suffering from malignant conditions such as lymphoma, leukaemia, Hodgkins disease or other tumours of the reticulo-endothelial system, or where the immunological mechanism may be impaired as in hypogammaglobulinaemia.
iv. Pregnant women, because of the theoretical risk of fetal infection. However if a pregnant woman must travel to a high-risk area, she should be vaccinated since the risk from yellow fever outweighs that of vaccination.
v. Persons known to be hypersensitive to neomycin, polymyxin, egg or chick protein. A letter stating that vaccination is contraindicated on these grounds may be acceptable in some countries. Advice should be sought from the Embassy.
vi. HIV positive individuals should NOT be given yellow fever vaccine. See Section 1.3.1.

18.5.2 If more than one live vaccine is required, they should either be given at the same time in different sites or with an interval of 3 weeks between them.

18.5.3 Infants under 9 months should only be vaccinated if the risk of yellow fever is unavoidable. (18.4.2)

18.6 There is no risk of transmission from imported cases since the mosquito vector does not occur in the UK.

18.7 Supplies

Manufactured and supplied by Wellcome, Tel. 0270 583151.

18.8 Bibliography

Fox JP, Cabral AS
The duration of immunity following vaccination with the 17D strain of yellow fever virus
Am. J. Hyg. 1943; 37; 93–120

Freestone DS et al
Stabilised 17D yellow fever vaccine: dose response studies, clinical reactions and effects on hepatic function
J. Biol Stand. 1977: 5(3), 181–6.

Groot H, Ribeivo RB
Neutralising and HAI antibody to yellow fever 17 years after vaccination with 17D vaccine
Bull WHO 1962; 27; 699–707

18.9 Yellow Fever Vaccination Centres: England

[A] Public centres
[B] Private centres open to members of the public
[C] Private centres which only serve the staff of the sponsoring organisation.

AYLESBURY [B]

RAF Institute of Pathology & Tropical Medicine
Halton
Aylesbury Bucks HP22 5PG

0296-623535

BARTON [B]

Dr DJ Sydenham
The Surgery
Hexton Road
Barton Beds MK45 4TA

0582-882050

BARROW-IN-FURNESS [B]

Vickers Limited Medical Department
5 Cavendish Park
Barrow-in-Furness
Cumbria LA14 2SE

0229-23366

BARNSLEY [A]

New Street Health Centre

0226-286122 ext 3100

BASINGSTOKE [A]

Basingstoke District Hospital
Outpatients Department

0256-473202 or 025671-286

BATH [B]

West England Wellcare Ltd
Medical Screening Centre
7 Great Pulteney Street
Bath BA2 4BR

0225-64231

BEDFORD [B]

Central Medical Systems Ltd
Rothesay House
Rothesay Place Bedford MK40 3PX

0234-271844

BIRMINGHAM [A]

90 Lancaster Street

021-235-3428

BLACKBURN [A]

Larkhill Health Centre

0254-63611 ext 231

BOLTON [B]

Newlands Medical Centre
Chorley New Road Bolton BL1 5BP

0204-40342/3

BOURNEMOUTH [A]

Avebury Child Health Clinic

0202-25253

BRADFORD [A]

Leeds Road Hospital

0274-729681 ext 45/58

BRIGHTON [A]

School Clinic
Morley Street

0273-693600 ext 271

BRISTOL [A]

Manulife House

0272-290666 ext 250

CAMBRIDGE [A]

Addenbrooke's Hospital

0223-245151 ext 7538

CANTERBURY [B]

The Chaucer Hospital
Nackington Road
Canterbury Kent CT4 7AR

0227 455466

CARLISLE [A]

The Central Clinic

0228-36451

CARTERTON (Oxfordshire) [B]

The Surgery
17 Alvescot Road
Carterton Oxfordshire OX8 3JL

0993-844567

CHEADLE [B]

AMI Alexandra Hospital
Mill Lane
Cheadle Cheshire SK8 2PX

061-428-3656

CHELMSFORD [A]

The Medical Centre
Ground Floor Block A
County Hall

0245-492211 ext 2756

COLCHESTER [B]

Priory House
St Botolph's Street
Colchester Essex CO2 7EA

0206-560050

COVENTRY [A]

Edyrean Walker Ward
Gulson Hospital
Gulson Road
Coventry CV1 2HR

0203-24055 ext 6035/6036

CROYDON [B]

The Executive Medical Centre
Canterbury House
Sydenham Road Croydon
Surrey CR0 2ls

01-688-3430

DERBY [A]

Cathedral Road Clinic

0332-45934

DONCASTER [A]

Chequer Road Health Clinic

0302-67051 ext 240

EXETER [A]

Dean Clarke House

0392-52211 ext 211

FELIXSTOWE [B]

Dr BMG Clarke
Central Surgery
201 Hamilton Road
Felixstowe Suffolk IP16 7DT

0392-283197

GATWICK [B]

British Caledonian Vaccination
Centre
South Terminal 3rd Floor
London (Gatwick) Airport
Horley Surrey LM6 0LH

0293-27890 ext 2351 or
0293-28822 ext 3593/3895

GLOUCESTER [A]

Gloucestershire Royal Hospital

0452-28555 ext 4210

GREAT MISSENDEN [B]

Chiltern Hospital
Great Missenden Buckinghamshire

02406-6565

GREAT YARMOUTH [B]

North Sea Medical Centre Ltd
3 Lowestoft Road
Gorleston-on-Sea
Great Yarmouth Norfolk NR31 6SG

0493-600011/663264

GRIMSBY [A]

The Clinic
0472-74111 ext 7890/7843

GUILDFORD [B]

The Robens Institute
Southern Counties Occupational
Health Service
University of Surrey Guildford
Surrey GU2 5XH

0483-509238

Yellow Fever

Immunisation against Infectious Disease

HARLOW [B]

Harlow Industrial Health Service
Edinburgh House
Edinburgh Way Harlow
Essex CM20 2DG

0279-22377

HARROW [B]

Harrow Health Care Centre
84–88 Pinner Road
Harrow Middlesex HA1 4LF

01-861-1221

HAVANT [B]

BUPA Hospital Bartons Road
Havant Hants PO9 5NP

0705-454511

HEATHROW [B]

British Airways Medical Service
Speedbird House Medical Centre
London (Heathrow) Airport
Hounslow Middlesex TW6 2JA

01-562-5453

HEATHROW [B]

British Airways Medical Service
Central Area Medical Department
(Queen's Building)
London (Heathrow) Airport
Hounslow Middlesex

01-562-7903

HULL [B]

Dr KJ Kutte
415 Beverley Road
Hull HU5 1LX

0482-42808

HULL [B]

University Health Service
University of Hull
187 Cottingham Road
Hull HU5 2EG

0482-46311

HULL [A]

The Central Clinic

0482-223191 ext 2272/2274

ILFORD [B]

The Surgery
150 Longwood Gardens
Clayhall Ilford
Essex IGE 0BE

01-550-6362

IPSWICH [B]

Orchard Street Health Centre
Ipswich Suffolk IP4 2PU

0473-213261

LANCASTER [A]

Ashton Road Clinic

0524-65944 ext 3717

LEEDS [A]

Halton Clinic

0532-486351

LEICESTER [A]

St Peter's Health Centre

0533-559600 ext 230

LINCOLN [A]

St Mark's House

0522-27196

LIVERPOOL [A]

International Vaccination Clinic
Sefton General Hospital

051-733-4020 ext 2202

LIVERPOOL [A]

School of Tropical Medicine

051-708-9393

LIVERPOOL [B]

General Council of British Shipping
Mann Island
Pier Head Liverpool L3 1DQ

051-236-6031

LONDON [A]

Yellow Fever Vaccination Service
Hospital for Tropical Diseases

01-387-4411 ext 136/137

LONDON [B]

Dr J Joseph
Amoco Europe Incorporated
48 Wimpole Street
London W1M 7BD

01-935-4357 or 01-486-7876

LONDON [B]

British Airways
Immunisation Medical Centre
75 Regents Street London W1

01-439-9584/5

LONDON [B]

Thomas Cook Group Limited
45 Berkeley Street
London W1A 1EB

01-499-4000

LONDON [B]

Dr C Goodson-Wickes
8 Devonshire Place
London W1N 1PB

01-935-5011

LONDON [B]

PPP Immunization Centre
99 New Cavendish Street
London W1M 7FQ

01-637-8941

LONDON [B]

West London Designated
Vaccinating Centre
53 Great Cumberland Place
London W1H 7LH

01-262-6456

LONDON [B]

Dr R Hart
4 Norfolk Place
London W2 1QN

01-723-7891

LONDON [B]

Trailfinders Travel Centre
Medical Advisory and Immunization
Centre
42 Earls Court Road
London W8 6EJ

01-938-3444

LONDON [B]

Dr MM Ferris
4 Frobisher House
Dolphin Square London SW1 3LN

01-798-8520

Yellow Fever

Yellow Fever

LONDON [B]

Dr C Goodson-Wickes
The Surgery
95a Jermyn Street
London SW1Y 6JE

01-930-2800

LONDON [B]

Dr IC Perry
19 Clivedon Place
London SW1 8HD

01-730-8045

LONDON [B]

Avicenna Clinic
6 Penywern Road
London SW5 9ST

01-370-7731/2 or 01-373-3196/7

LONDON [B]

Cromwell Hospital
Cromwell Road
London SW5 0TU

01-370-4233

LONDON [B]

Mildmay Mission Hospital
Hackney Road
London E2 7NA

01-739-2331

LONDON [B]

Dr Gill & partners
23 Lawrence Lane
London EC2V 8DA

01-606-6159

LONDON [B]

Dr HMJ Kindness
65 London Wall
London EC2M 7AD

01-638-3001

LONDON [B]

Dr Brackenridge & partners
3 Lombard Street
London EC3V 9AL

01-626-6985

LONDON [B]

Dr Hugh Richards
4 Mitre Court Chambers
4 Old Mitre Court
Fleet Street
London EC4Y 7BP

01-353-4151

LONDON [B]

The Medical Department
Unilever House
Blackfriars Embankment
London EC4 P4BQ

01-822-6017

LONDON [B]

BUPA Medical Centre
Webb House
210 Pentonville Road
King's Cross
London NW1 9TA

01-837-8641

LUTON [B]

The Surgery
163 Dunstable Road
Luton LU1 1BW

0582-23553/5

MAIDSTONE [A]
Springfield
0622-671411 ext 2726

MANCHESTER [A]
Town Hall Extension
061-234-4921/4932

MANCHESTER [B]
British Airways Immunization Centre
Market Street
Manchester
061-831-7161

MANCHESTER [B]
Airport Medical Centre
Manchester Airport PLC
Manchester M22 5PA
061-489-3000

MIDDLESBROUGH [A]
West Lane Hospital
0642-813144 ext 265

MILTON KEYNES [B]
Milton Keynes Occupational Health Service Ltd
Whalley Drive
Bletchley
Milton Keynes MK3 6EN
0908-75194/5

NEWCASTLE UPON TYNE [A]
Shieldfield Health and Social Services Centre
091-273-8811 ext 22666

NEWPORT Isle of Wight [A]
St Mary's Hospital
0983-524081 ext 4209

NORTHAMPTON [A]
St Giles Street Clinic
0604-37221

NORWICH [A]
West Pottergate Health Centre
0603-620263

NOTTINGHAM [A]
Meadows Health Centre
0602-415333 ext 209

OXFORD [A]
Community Health Offices
Radcliffe Infirmary
0865-249891 ext 4816

PAIGNTON [B]
The Clinic
Midvale Road
Paignton Devon
0803-522762

PENZANCE [A]
Health Clinic
Bellair
0736-62321

PLYMOUTH [A]
Longfield House
0752-834598

Yellow Fever

Immunisation against Infectious Disease 107

Yellow Fever

PORTSMOUTH [A]
Battenburg Avenue Clinic
0705-664235

RADLETT [B]
The Red House
124 Watling Street
Radlett Herts WD7 7JQ
09276-5606

REDBRIDGE [B]
The Roding Hospital
Roding Lane South
Redbridge Essex IG4 5PZ
01-551-1100

RICHMOND (Surrey) [A]
King's Road Clinic
01-940-9879

SHEFFIELD [A]
Mulberry Street
0742-768885 ext 157

SHREWSBURY [A]
Cross Houses
0743-75242 ext 386

SLOUGH [B]
The Nuffield Hospital
Wexham Street
Slough
Berkshire SL3 6NH
02816-2999

SOUTHAMPTON [A]
Cunard Steamship Company PLC
South Western House
Canute Road Southampton
Hampshire SO9 1ZA
0703-229933 ext 366

SOUTHAMPTON [A]
General Council of British Shipping
19–23 Canute Road
Southampton SO1 1FJ
0703-223546

SOUTHAMPTON [A]
Central Health Clinic
0703-634321 ext 235/265

SOUTHEND-ON-SEA [A]
Queensway House
0702-616322 ext 213

SOUTH SHIELDS [B]
General Council of British Shipping
5 Cornwallis Street
South Shields
Tyne & Wear NE33 1BB
0632-563172

TAUNTON [A]
County Hall
0823-73491 ext 245/255

TILBURY [B]
The Health Centre
London Road
Tilbury Essex
03752-2028

Immunisation against Infectious Disease

TRING [B]

The Surgery
23 High Street
Tring Herts HP23 5AS

044282-2468

TRURO [A]

District Health Office

0872-72202

TWYFORD [B]

The Surgery
Loddon Hall Road
Twyford Berkshire RG10 9JA

0734-340112

WEST BROMWICH [B]

Midlands Occupational Health
Service Ltd
83 Birmingham Road
West Bromwich
West Midlands B70 1PX

021-553-7116/9

WHITBY [B]

Whitby Group Practice
The Health Centre
Whitby Hospital Whitby
North Yorkshire YO21 1DP

0947-602828

WORCESTER PARK (Surrey) [A]

Manor Drive Clinic

01-337-0246

YORK [A]

Monkgate Health Centre

0904-30351 ext 19

SCOTLAND

ABERDEEN [A]

View Terrace Clinic

0224-631633

ARRAN [A]

Ayrshire General Hospital
Irvine

0294-74191

DUNDEE [A]

King's Cross Hospital

0382-816116 ext 224

EDINBURGH [A]

15–17 Carlton Terrace

031-557-2100

GLASGOW [A]

20 Cochrane Street

041-227-4411

ORKNEY [A]

Orkney Health Board

0856-2763 ext 257

SHETLAND [A]

Gilbert Bain Hospital

0595-5678

WALES

CARDIFF [A]

St David's Hospital

0222-372451 ext 2662/2669

Yellow Fever

HAVERFORDWEST [A]
Community Health Clinic
Merlins Hill
0437-67801 ext 251

LLANDUDNO [A]
Aberconwy Community Office
0492-860011

NEWPORT (Gwent) [A]
Clytha Clinic
Clytha Park Road
0633-64011

SWANSEA [A]
Swansea Central Clinic
0792-51501 ext 303

NORTHERN IRELAND

BALLYMENA [A]
51 Castle Street
0266-56324/2108/55160

BELFAST [A]
Lincoln Avenue Clinic
0232-748363

OMAGH [A]
The Health Centre
0662-3521 ext 263

ISLE OF MAN

DOUGLAS [A]
Noble's Hospital
0624-73661 ext 279

19 Appendix: Immunoglobulin

19.1 Introduction

19.1.1 Injection of human immunoglobulin produces immediate passive immunity lasting a few weeks. There are two types:

i) Human normal immunoglobulin (HNIG) is derived from the pooled plasma of blood donors. HNIG contains antibody to measles, mumps, varicella, hepatitis A and other viruses which are currently prevalent in the general population.

ii) Specific immunoglobulins for varicella, tetanus, rabies and hepatitis B. These are obtained from the pooled blood of convalescent patients or donors recently immunised with the relevant vaccine.

All immunoglobulins are obtained from HIV negative blood donations.

19.2 Human Normal Immunoglobulin (HNIG)

This is available in 1.7ml ampoules containing 250mg, and 5ml ampoules containing 750mg. It is given by intramuscular injection except where specifically stated that it is for intravenous injection. It should be stored at 0–4°C; the expiry date given on the packet must be observed.

Recommendations for its use are given in the relevant Sections.

19.2.1 *Measles (Section 7)*

HNIG

For prophylaxis in children at special risk, to be given as soon as possible after contact with measles. Such children include those with compromised immunity, and those with recent severe illness for whom measles should be avoided.

To prevent an attack:

Age	Dose
Under 1 year	250mg
1–2 years	500mg
3 and over	750mg

Immunisation against Infectious Disease

To allow an attenuated attack:

	Under 1 year	100mg
	1 year or over	250mg

NB This preparation must NOT be used with measles vaccine. An interval of at least 3 months should be observed between an injection of immunoglobulin and subsequent measles vaccination.

19.2.2 *Rubella (Section 9)*

Immunoglobulin after exposure does NOT prevent infection in non-immune contacts and is NOT recommended for protection of pregnant women exposed to rubella. It may however reduce the likelihood of a clinical attack; it should be given as soon as possible after exposure when termination of pregnancy would be unacceptable. Serological follow-up of recipients is essential.

Dose. 750mg

19.2.3 *Hepatitis A (Section 12.9)*

a) To control outbreaks – close contacts of all ages.

Under 10 years	250mg
Ten years and over	500mg

b) For travellers abroad to all countries excluding Europe, N America, Australia and New Zealand.

Period abroad	Age	Dose
2 months or less;	Under 10 years	125mg
	Ten years and over	250mg
3–5 months;	Under 10 years	250mg
	Ten years and over	500mg

NB HNIG may interfere with the immune response to live virus vaccines which should therefore be given at least 3 weeks before or three months after an injection of HNIG. This does not apply to yellow fever vaccine since HNIG does not contain antibody to this virus. For travellers, if there is insufficient time, the recommended interval may have to be ignored.

19.2.4 *Mumps*

HNIG contains mumps antibody and can be used for post-exposure protection although its value is uncertain. Mumps-specific immunoglobulin is no longer available.

Dose		
	0–5 years	250mg
	6–10 years	500mg
	11–14 years	750mg
	15 +	1000mg

19.2.5 *Supplies*

NHIG: From Central Public Health Laboratory Tel: 01 200 6868 (CDSC)
Public Health Laboratories, England and Wales
Blood Transfusion Service, Scotland
Blood Products Laboratory Tel. 01 953 6191

Immuno Tel. 0732 458101 (Gammabulin)
Kabivitrum Tel. 0895 51144 (Kabiglobulin)

For intravenous use:
Cutter Tel. 02814 5151 (Gamimune-N)
Biotest UK Tel. 021 733 3393 (Intraglobin)
Sandoz Tel. 01 890 1366 (Sandoglobulin)

19.3 Specific Immunoglobulins

19.3.1 *Tetanus (Section 5)*

A specific anti-tetanus immunoglobulin is available for the immediate treatment of tetanus-prone wounds in the following individuals:–

a) Unimmunised.
b) Immunisation history unknown
c) Over 10 years since last tetanus vaccine

Available in 1ml ampoules containing 250 IU.

Dose. Prevention: 250 IU, or 500 IU if more than 24 hours have elapsed since injury, or there is a risk of heavy contamination.
Treatment: 30–300 IU/kg given in multiple sites.

Supplies
Regional Blood Transfusion Centres
Wellcome Tel. 0270 583151 (Humotet)

19.3.2 *Hepatitis B (Section 12)*
Specific immunoglobulin (HBIG) is available for passive protection against hepatitis B (See 12.8).
Available in 1ml ampoules containing 100IU, and 5ml ampoules containing 500IU for intramuscular injection.

Dose:

ADULTS:– 500 IU (5ml) preferably within 48 hours and not more than 10 days after exposure. A second dose 4 weeks later is required unless:

    a) There is evidence of past HBV infection in the recipie it's pre-immunoglobulin blood sample, or
    b) Tests show that the inoculum is anti-HBe positive and therefore not infective, or
    c) A course of HB vaccine is begun at the same time as the first dose of HBIG is given.

NEWBORN:– initial dose; 200 IU as soon as possible and within 48 hours of birth.

Subsequent doses;
    a) For infants of high-risk carrier mothers (12.3.5): no further HBIG if HB vaccine is given at the same time as the first dose. If HB vaccine is delayed, 2nd dose of HBIG 100 IU is given one month later.
    b) For infants of mothers with acute hepatitis B: passive/active immunisation as for a).

NOTES.

1. HBIG is not appropriate for treatment of any type of hepatitis B infection.

2. It is not available for travellers.

3. A blood sample should be collected before HBIG is given but administration should not be delayed until test result is known.

4. HBIG will NOT inhibit the antibody response when given at same time as HB vaccine.

Supplies
Central Public Health Laboratory Tel. 01 200 6868
(Hepatitis Epidemiology Unit)
Public Health Laboratories
Scotland: Blood Transfusion Service (see 13.8.3)

If HBIG is ordered from sources other than the Hepatitis Epidemiology Unit, it should be reported to the HEU as soon as possible by whoever places the order.

19.3.3 *Rabies specific immunoglobulin (HRIG)*

HRIG is used after exposure to rabies to provide rapid protection until rabies vaccine, which should be given at the same time, becomes effective. Details of treatment are given in Section 13. HRIG is available in 1ml ampoules containing 500 IU.

Dose. 20 IU/kg body weight. Up to half the dose is infiltrated in and around the wound after thorough cleansing and the rest given by intramuscular injection.

Supplies
Central Public Health Laboratory, Tel. 01 200 6868
   (Virus Reference Laboratory)

19.3.4 *Anti-varicella-zoster immunoglobulin (ZIG)*

ZIG is available in 1.7ml ampoules containing 250mg for intramuscular injection and is recommended for the following:

1. Immunosuppressed and leukaemic contacts of chicken pox or herpes zoster.
2. Individuals with debilitating disease who are in contact with chicken pox or herpes zoster.
3. Neonates born 6 days or less after onset of maternal chicken pox.
4. Neonates whose mothers develop chicken pox after delivery.
5. Neonates in contact with chicken pox or zoster whose mothers have no history of chicken pox.
6. Pregnant contacts.

Immunisation against Infectious Disease

7. Treatment of a serious attack. (There is no evidence that ZIG is of value but it is occasionally used if it can be given within a few days of onset).

Dose (for prevention and treatment):

0–5 years	250mg
6–10 years	500mg
11–14 years	750mg
15 +	1000mg

19.3.5 Notes.

1. ZIG does not prevent infection even when given within 72 hours of exposure. It may attenuate an attack if given up to 10 days after exposure. Both sub-clinical and clinical attacks occur; the latter are occasionally severe despite ZIG.

2. In the event of a second exposure more than 3 weeks after ZIG is given, a further dose will be required.

3. Immunosuppressed and leukaemic contacts

    a. With the exception of bone marrow transplant recipients, immunosuppressed patients with a history of chicken pox do not require ZIG.

    b. Patients with a history of chicken pox who are at long-term risk (e.g. following transplant) should be tested for V-Z antibody by an appropriate test. Many will have antibody and will not require ZIG should future exposure occur.

4. Neonatal and pregnant contacts

    a. Neonatal varicella can still occur despite ZIG prophylaxis. Infection is usually mild but rare cases of fatal varicella have been reported in neonates who have received ZIG.

    b. In the following neonates maternal antibody will be present and ZIG is not required:–
    i) Infants born more than 6 days AFTER maternal chicken pox.
    ii) Infants whose mothers have a history of chicken pox.
    iii) Infants whose mothers develop ZOSTER before or after delivery.

    c. Premature infants born before 30 weeks gestation or with birth weight below 1kg may not possess maternal antibody despite a positive history in the mother.

d. The main indication for ZIG prophylaxis in pregnant contacts is prevention of severe maternal infection; fetal damage is rare.

e. Pregnant contacts should be tested for V-Z antibody before ZIG is given since about two-thirds of women are immune despite a negative history.

Supplies
Central Public Health Laboratory Tel. 01 200 6868.
 (CDSC)

19.4 Antivaccinia immunoglobulin

Information and supplies from Virus Reference Laboratory, Public Health Laboratory Service. Tel. 01 200 4400.